T0259523

Research

Guest Editor

ROBIN D. FROMAN, RN, PhD, FAAN

PERIOPERATIVE NURSING CLINICS

www.periopnursing.theclinics.com

Consulting Editor
NANCY GIRARD, PhD, RN, FAAN

September 2009 • Volume 4 • Number 3

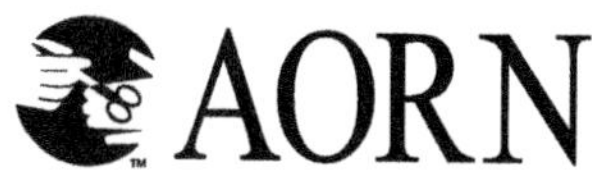

SAUNDERS an imprint of ELSEVIER, Inc.

W.B. SAUNDERS COMPANY

A Division of Elsevier Inc.

1600 John F. Kennedy Boulevard • Suite 1800 • Philadelphia, Pennsylvania 19103-2899

http://www.periopnursing.theclinics.com

PERIOPERATIVE NURSING CLINICS Volume 4, Number 3

September 2009 ISSN 1556-7931, ISBN-13: 978-1-4377-1261-2, ISBN-10: 1-4377-1261-4

Editor: Katie Hartner
Developmental Editor: Donald Mumford

Perioperative Nursing Clinics (ISSN 1556-7931) is published quarterly by Elsevier, 360 Park Avenue South, New York, NY 10010. Months of issue are March, June, September and December. Business and Editorial Offices: 1600 John F. Kennedy Blvd., Suite 1800, Philadelphia, PA 19103-2899. Customer Service Office: 11830 Westline Industrial Drive, St. Louis, MO 63146. Periodicals postage paid at New York, NY and at additional mailing offices. Subscription prices are $116.00 per year (domestic individuals), $209.00 per year (domestic institutions), $58.00 per year (domestic students/residents), $116.00 per year (Canadian individuals), $240.00 per year (Canadian institutions), $150 per year (international individuals), $240 per year (international institutions), and $62.00 per year (International and Canadian students/residents). Foreign air speed delivery is included in all *Clinics* subscription prices. All prices are subject to change without notice. **POSTMASTER:** Send change of address to *Perioperative Nursing Clinics*, Customer Service (orders, claims, online, change of address): Elsevier Periodicals Customer Service, 11830 Westline Industrial Drive, St. Louis, MO 63146. Tel: 1-800-654-2452 (U.S. and Canada). Fax: 314-523-5170. E-mail: journalscustomerservice-usa@elsevier.com (for print support); journalsonlinesupport-usa@elsevier.com (for online support).

Reprints. For copies of 100 or more, of articles in this publication, please contact the Commercial Rights Department, Elsevier Inc., 360 Park Avenue South, New York, NY 10010-1710; phone: (+1) 212-633-3813; fax: (+1) 212-462-1935; e-mail: reprints@elsevier.com.

Printed and bound by CPI Group (UK) Ltd, Croydon, CR0 4YY

Transferred to Digital Print 2012

Contributors

CONSULTING EDITOR

NANCY GIRARD, PhD, RN, FAAN
Consultant, Boerne; Clinical Associate Professor, Acute Nursing Care Department, University of Texas Health Science Center, San Antonio, Texas

GUEST EDITOR

ROBIN D. FROMAN, RN, PhD, FAAN
Interim Director, Center for Nursing Scholarship, School of Nursing, University of Connecticut, Storrs, Connecticut

AUTHORS

LYDA C. ARÉVALO-FLECHAS, RN, PhD
Clinical Assistant Professor, Department of Acute Nursing Care, The University of Texas Health Science Center, San Antonio School of Nursing; and John A. Hartford Foundation, Claire M. Fagin Fellow, San Antonio, Texas

KAY C. AVANT, RN, PhD, FAAN
Zeller Professor and Chair, Family Nursing Department, University of Texas Health Science Center at San Antonio, San Antonio, Texas

CHERYL TATANO BECK, DNSc, CNM, FAAN
Distinguished Professor, School of Nursing, University of Connecticut, Storrs, Connecticut

ROBIN D. FROMAN, RN, PhD, FAAN
Interim Director, Center for Nursing Scholarship, School of Nursing, University of Connecticut, Storrs, Connecticut

NANCY GIRARD, PhD, RN, FAAN
Consultant, Boerne; Clinical Associate Professor, Acute Nursing Care Department, University of Texas Health Science Center, San Antonio, Texas

BARBARA J. HOLTZCLAW, PhD, RN, FAAN
Professor, Graduate Program Associate Director, Translational Science, Donald W. Reynolds Center of Geriatric Nursing Excellence, College of Nursing, University of Oklahoma Health Science Center, Norman, Oklahoma

CHERYL A. LEHMAN, PhD, RN, CNS
Associate Professor/Clinical, The University of Texas Health Science Center at San Antonio, School of Nursing, Acute Nursing Department, San Antonio, Texas

SHARON L. LEWIS, RN, PhD, FAAN
Professor Schools of Nursing and Medicine, University of Texas Health Science Center at San Antonio; and Clinical Nurse Scientist, South Texas Veterans Health Care System, San Antonio, Texas

KAREN MENESES, PhD, RN, FAAN
Professor and Associate Dean for Research, School of Nursing, University of Alabama at Birmingham, Birmingham, Alabama

STEVEN V. OWEN, PhD
University Professor Emeritus, University of Connecticut, Storrs, Connecticut

CATHY ROCHE, BSN, RN, FAAN
Doctoral Student, School of Nursing, University of Alabama at Birmingham, Birmingham, Alabama

Contents

Preface ix

Robin D. Froman

Reading and Interpreting a Quantitative Research Study 201

Barbara J. Holtzclaw

Nurse clinicians make hundreds of small decisions every hour based on training, experience, and logical problem solving. Experience-based knowledge develops as they begin noticing cause-and-effect relationships and form personal theories that make them highly attentive to some factors and suspicious about others. The expert clinician uses these heightened clues about relationships to predict and avoid problems. Quantitative research provides the clinician with other information, gathered in a far more formal way, using sensitive measurements and controls to account for factors that have competing influence. This article offers pointers and a roadmap for reading and interpreting the formalized language, structure, and outcomes of quantitative research reports, with emphasis on issues of validity that affect a study's strength for evidence-based practice decisions.

Viewing the Rich, Diverse Landscape of Qualitative Research 217

Cheryl Tatano Beck

Qualitative research stems from the naturalistic paradigm. In this article, six of the most common qualitative research designs are discussed: phenomenology, grounded theory, ethnography, historical research, narrative analysis, and meta-synthesis. Some of these research designs are illustrated by concrete examples from the author's research program on postpartum mood and anxiety disorders, and others are examples from published studies in perioperative nursing. The article ends with a discussion of criteria to assess the rigor of qualitative research.

Reading and Evaluating Theory in a Research Publication 231

Kay C. Avant

This article explains how theory is used in quantitative and qualitative research reports. Several confusing concepts are defined and clarified. Questions are posed to help readers determine whether theory was used correctly in the various types of research reports. The article will help the reader evaluate the state of the theory and whether it is appropriate for use in informing practice.

Quality Measurement as the Cornerstone of Respectable Research 237

Robin D. Froman

Research studies, regardless of whether they are qualitative, quantitative, or mixed methodology, are based upon data. These data represent things that have been measured, either objectively or subjectively. These foundational data create the basis for statistical analysis, hypothesis testing, interpretation of themes, or development of theories about phenomena. As such, the measured data are the underpinning for research studies and are potentially the Achilles' heel of the studies. This article discusses types of reliability estimation and validity estimation, pointing the way to better research methods.

Making Sense of Published Statistics 245

Steven V. Owen

Readers of quantitative research are often put off by the mysteries of statistical jargon. This article introduces, simplifies, and explains common terms of statistical language. The case is also made that authors of quantitative research should strive to balance statistical significance with clinical significance. Clinical significance may be assessed by effect sizes, which are widespread in some professions, but remain underreported in the health professions.

Recruitment and Retention in Clinical Research 259

Karen Meneses and Cathy Roche

Recruitment is defined as the process of identifying and enrolling volunteers for participation in a research study. Retention is the ability to maintain individual participation throughout the duration of the research study. Recruitment and retention are enormously vital aspects of clinical research. This article reviews the process of identifying and enrolling participants for recruitment; describes regulatory requirements influencing subject recruitment; discusses special considerations in the recruitment of children, minorities, and at risk individuals; describes the process of participant retention; describes the utility of tracking databases; and explores clinical nursing roles and responsibilities in recruitment and retention in clinical research.

Practical Issues in Conducting Hospital-based Research 269

Cheryl A. Lehman

Conducting research in the hospital setting presents unique challenges. These include the challenges and opportunities in being an "insider" or an "outsider" in the clinical setting. This article offers an overview of these challenges and suggests ways that the researcher might overcome them.

Bridging the Gap Between Research and Clinical Practice 277

Sharon L. Lewis

Nurses need to use research findings to develop enhanced assessment skills, revise policies and procedures, and develop effective interventions so that research findings will translate to improved patient outcomes. The primary purposes of this article are (1) to identify barriers to using research in clinical practice and (2) to discuss effective ways to facilitate integration of research findings in clinical practice.

Beyond Translated Consents: Culturally Competent Research **287**

Lyda C. Arévalo-Flechas

Racial and ethnic minorities, now roughly one third of the US population, are expected to become the majority in 2042. Although the US population at large enjoyed longer lives and improved health during the latter part of the twentieth century, racial and ethnic minorities experienced striking health disparities. Mitigation of health disparities can be achieved, in part, by the delivery of culturally competent health care. The quest for the knowledge necessary to achieve culturally competent care starts with the inclusion of racial and ethnic minorities in research studies that are culturally competent. This article provides an overview of the stages in the Cross continuum of cultural competency and describes Meleis' eight cultural competence guidelines for research.

Dissemination of Findings: The Final Step of Investigation **297**

Nancy Girard

This article focuses on the final step of research and clinical study, which is the dissemination of findings. It is mandated that the findings of empiric and discovery research be published to build on a body of knowledge to further nursing theory and to improve patient care. Quality improvement projects in the clinical area are as important as research for improving care and should also be shared with colleagues. The preparation of manuscripts for each is described, as well as tips on writing and submitting manuscripts.

Index **307**

FORTHCOMING ISSUES

December 2009

Pain, Analgesia and Anesthesia
Valerie Girard-Powell, RN,
Guest Editor

March 2010

Surgical Instruments
Katherine Gaberson, PhD, RN, CNOR,
Guest Editor

June 2010

Radiology
Kathleen Gross, MSN, RN, BVC, CRN,
Guest Editor

RECENT ISSUES

June 2009

Education
Jane C. Rothrock, DNSc, RN, CNOR, FAAN,
Guest Editor

March 2009

Leadership
Nancy Girard, PhD, RN, FAAN,
Guest Editor

December 2008

Patient Safety
Donna S. Watson, RN, MSN, CNOR,
ARNP-BC, *Guest Editor*

Preface

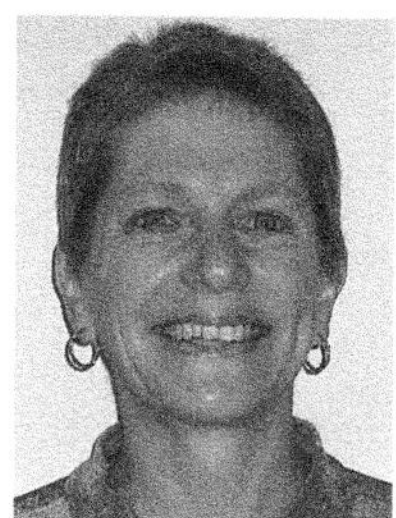

Robin D. Froman, RN, PhD, FAAN
Guest Editor

This issue of *Perioperative Nursing Clinics* is unusual for a number of reasons. As the issue's Guest Editor I would like to use this Preface to outline the issue's unique characteristics and explain why it was compiled in this manner.

First, all of the authors contributing to the issue know each other, and many have co-authored articles previously. It has been my great fortune to have worked with each one of these authors and my delight to count each as a personal friend. The familiarity we all share provides a foundation of mutual respect and appreciation of each other's work, which is reflected in this issue. This characteristic also allows the authors of each article to refer meaningfully to the others' writing within the volume, weaving context among the articles rather than having distinct article boundaries. In short, the articles create integrated content throughout the issue instead of being just a collection of stand-alone articles.

This leads to the second unique aspect of the issue. Taken together, the articles add up to a sum that is greater than their parts. Cross-referencing throughout the articles contributes to that, but a greater driving force was the discussions Dr. Nancy Girard and I had in conceptualizing the issue. As a seasoned perioperative nurse, Dr. Girard is sensitive to the needs of practicing nurses. She approached me to edit this issue with the intent that it could be used by practicing nurses as a research primer. Unfortunately, most contemporary research texts are constructed for use in a college course, not by individual nurses or for use in practice settings. Our goal in writing these articles was to provide abundant practice examples with which clinicians—not just students—could connect. We also wanted the articles to add up to an easily accessible introduction to the research process.

The third unique element of this issue is that three of the authors are former students of one or more of the authors represented herein. The entire issue reflects evolution and development from learner to independent scholar. In some cases, the student role was completed many years ago, in others it was completed just recently. Additionally, all of the authors can be considered credible and productive researchers; they have all received competitive grant funds, more often large federal grants. Furthermore, many have sat on National Institutes of Health study sections as grant proposal reviewers.

Perioperative Nursing Clinics 4 (2009) ix–x
doi:10.1016/j.cpen.2009.05.011
periopnursing.theclinics.com
1556-7931/09/$ – see front matter

Finally, the roster of authors represents a wide range of age, location of educational institution and residence, practice concentration, ethnicity, and gender. The authors and I are diverse in our backgrounds and what we bring to these articles. However, we all share in the hope that you will enjoy reading this issue, and that it will offer some fresh ideas you can use in your own research endeavors. We had fun creating this issue of the *Clinics* and hope you will feel some of that enthusiasm while reading.

Robin D. Froman, RN, PhD, FAAN
Center for Nursing Scholarship
School of Nursing
University of Connecticut
Storrs, CT 06268, USA

E-mail address:
rdf@vbbn.com (R.D. Froman)

Reading and Interpreting a Quantitative Research Study

Barbara J. Holtzclaw, PhD, RN, FAAN

KEYWORDS

- Quantitative research • Descriptive designs • Experiments
- Quasi-experiments • Clinical trials

Perhaps you have noticed a growing trend to include research articles in all nursing publications, but particularly in clinical journals. This trend is, in part, a happy consequence of nurse clinicians embracing evidence-based practice and recognizing the need to base more of their current practice on sound evidence from research.[1] Examples incorporating best evidence are seen in published guidelines appearing in journals of the American Operating Room Association and the American Society of PeriAnesthesia Nurses.[2–5] A large number of research articles published in clinical practice journals are in a category commonly called "quantitative research" because tests of interventions and clinical predictors fall into this category. Although nearly every nurse can enjoy reading a research article's introduction, justification of need for the study, and review of the current literature on a topic, the reader's attention often grows dim when reaching the methods section. It is tempting to jump to the end of the article to see how the author explains the study's outcome. This article is designed to nudge nurse clinicians to probe a little more deeply into the research evidence they read by equipping them with clues for interpreting the strengths or potential weaknesses that reside within the methods section. The focus is on factors that affect how a quantitative study is designed and controls are used to reduce error, how and why a study sample is chosen with such care, and to what extent these decisions affect the strength of the evidence. Although this brief article could not possibly substitute for a research textbook or course in quantitative research, information has been drawn from both of these sources with relevancy and application for the nurse in clinical practice in mind.

Donald W. Reynolds Center of Geriatric Nursing Excellence, College of Nursing, University of Oklahoma Health Science Center, 1100 North Stonewall, PO Box 26901, Oklahoma City, OK 73190, USA

E-mail address: bholtzcl@ouhsc.edu

Perioperative Nursing Clinics 4 (2009) 201–215
doi:10.1016/j.cpen.2009.05.005
periopnursing.theclinics.com

WHAT'S IN A NAME: DOES QUANTITATIVE IMPLY SOMETHING SPECIFIC?

The selection of a particular research method should be guided by the research question one has in mind and the most effective way to answer that question. As the name suggests, "quantitative" approaches are designed to help answer questions that can be answered by measuring quantifiable data, or data that can be represented by numerical characteristics. They are ideally suited for numerically describing things, phenomena, or conditions and for studying relationships between variables. Quantitative approaches are used to test hypotheses, to identify numerical differences between groups, or to quantify changes. Quantitative approaches are good choices for testing intervention effects and determining conditions associated with bad or good clinical outcomes. One should avoid the misconception that quantitative research is reserved for directly observable physiologic or behavioral variables. Numerous scales, inventories, and measurement methods that indirectly, but numerically, quantify feelings, perceptions, traits, and states are frequently used in quantitative research. For example, visual analogue scales are used to record the occurrence and intensity of pain by having the patient give a rating on a "ruler" and then converting the rating to quantitative data that can be analyzed statistically.

DETERMINING WHETHER A STUDY IS QUANTITATIVE

Not all quantitative research reports are identified explicitly by that descriptor. In fact, an article may be described by its design. A study may be described broadly as a descriptive (observational), experimental, or quasi-experimental study, or perhaps with one or more of its statistical perspectives, such as a comparative, correlational, or repeated measures study (eg, a quasi-experimental, comparative design, with repeated measures). Take a look at the research question and the way the study variables are described and measured. If the descriptors involve measurement in numbers or variables with numerical values assigned to them, and if the methods are designed to draw conclusions based on counting, correlating, comparing, or otherwise statistically analyzing those numbers, this is a quantitative study. Descriptive or observational studies are quantitative if they observe, quantify, and even seek relationships between variables but make no attempt to manipulate behaviors or conditions. Examples include studying the outcomes related to hospital and unit census reports, incidents related to staff-patient ratios, and staphylococcus infections related to patient age. Numerous clinical research studies have used this method to draw comparisons between treatment modalities and outcomes. Examples include studying the birth outcomes of hospital versus home born infants and comparing perineal muscle strength and incontinence in postpartum women with and without episiotomy. Although treatments or interventions were not assigned to the patient as a part of these studies, and although they are not actual experiments, they can provide inferential evidence that can suggest the influence of certain conditions or treatments. These descriptive studies often precede or lead to intervention studies. When descriptive studies use inferential statistics to infer attributes about a larger population from information drawn from a sample, they do not have the strength of evidence of an experiment because they cannot demonstrate cause. Nevertheless, these studies provide informative relational descriptions of clinical factors that bear watching or that need to be studied further while controlling for other possible explanations. Nurse researchers have for years generated important clinical hypotheses from descriptive studies that provided preliminary steps to later experimental work.

Experimental studies measure changes in quantities that occur after a treatment or intervention. These studies are done to examine cause and effect and often require procedures with repeated measures to compare a before and after change. Examples in nursing and health care include clinical trials, intervention studies, and pre- and posttests studying the effects of educational programs. Four factors make a study a true experiment: (1) randomized selection under control of the researcher of participants in the sample, (2) randomized assignment under the control of the researcher to treatment or control groups, (3) researcher control of the treatment (independent variable), and (4) control of the surrounding experimental condition. The operative word throughout is *control*, and in most human situations, particularly in clinical conditions, this is difficult or impossible to manage completely. The condition of random sampling means that every individual in the population under study would have an equal chance of being selected for a study. This condition is difficult when studying an unpredictable phenomenon such as shivering or postoperative fever. Once a sample is selected, randomization is required in assignment to treatment and control (comparison) groups. The ethical right for potential participants to not participate in or drop out of studies complicates true random representation of everyone in the population and achievement of random assignment. Control of assignment to comparative groups means the participants do not get to self-select to group membership or to drop out once they are assigned if they do not like the group they are in. Clearly, given ethical considerations, participants cannot be coerced to remain in their randomly assigned group; therefore, securing random assignment through the entire course of a study is difficult. It is also possible to have random selection of the sample without random assignment, or to have nonrandom selection but still exert random assignment to groups. These two "randoms" can function independently. Control of the treatment or experimental variable is a little more manageable than randomization. Drug trials are examples in which the treatment can be carefully controlled and "blinded" to the recipient and caregivers so that neither is aware of whether the recipients are in the treatment or control group. Control of the experimental conditions is most likely if the experiment is conducted in a laboratory or area that is consistent and free from extraneous stimuli. A sleep laboratory is an example of a controlled environment where effects of environmental temperature or humidity on sleep quality could be studied.

Quasi-experimental studies are also done to examine cause and effect but are performed in situations in which all of the criteria of true experimental control are not possible to exert. The quasi-experimental design was described by Campbell and Stanley in the early 1960s as a common way to examine causality in social science situations that could not be completely controlled. Quasi-experimental designs control as many threats to validity as possible.[6] Creating cause-and-effect inferences from quasi-experimental studies draws considerable criticism from research methodologists and statistical scientists when compared with controlled experimental designs.[7] Nevertheless, clinicians argue that the methodology is valuable in the numerous situations in health care in which complete randomization and control are not possible. Proponents insist that these studies often suggest causes that pave the way for more soundly based research ideas and more convincing causal links between interventions and outcomes.[8] An example of a quasi-experiment is a study performed by nurses on a surgical unit in a hospital in which patients received patient-controlled analgesia.[9] The study participants were assigned, but without randomization, to an experimental or control group to test the effects of a treatment intervention of multimedia education on pain management of postsurgical patients. The use of the patient-controlled analgesia was already prescribed by physicians. The environmental conditions surrounding the study were not controlled, but the outcome determined whether the structured multimedia educational intervention was as effective as or better than the traditional nurse-delivered instructions and pamphlets given to patients. The study results showed that the multimedia approach brought significantly higher improvement in pain relief in the treatment group. One could argue that there were differences between the groups that were not balanced by randomization. To warrant a change in standards for clinical practice or widespread use of economic, social, or health-related consequences, the quasi-experimental study requires replication and more rigorous testing; however, such unit-based studies continue to provide stronger direction for evidence-based practice than simple tradition or common sense. The quasi-experiment moves an idea from a purely descriptive one about relationships that bear watching to one that can be studied by controlling the type or conditions of a treatment and systematically measuring outcomes.

Because quantitative research includes highly controlled experimental studies and clinical trials that give best evidence of intervention outcomes, it has enjoyed a valued place in medical decision making. Movements in acute and critical care nursing have leaned toward evidence-based classifications based on a hierarchy of scientific "rigor" introduced by medicine and the Cochrane Collaboration in which the randomized clinical trial (RCT) was deemed the most appropriate; however, in medical and nursing care, there is recognition that an integration of research findings provides even better evidence. Polit and Beck provide a seven-level hierarchy that posits (1) systematic reviews of RCT and (2) systematic reviews of nonrandomized (quasi-experimental) clinical trials, in that order, above a single RCT as best evidence for clinical decisions.[10] Because patient comfort and subjective information are used in clinical decision making, quantitative research findings must also be balanced with qualitative input and clinical judgment. The fact that these aspects are considered in lower levels of evidence of intervention effectiveness does not negate their value but, rather, acknowledges the difficulty in controlling for an alternate explanation.

UNDERSTANDING TERMS USED IN RESEARCH ARTICLES

One thing that often puts off the clinician from reading quantitative research reports is an unfamiliarity or misunderstanding of the terms used. This observation is particularly true of the sections reporting the statistical findings, explaining why an entire article in this publication has been devoted to statistical issues. Even if one has learned research terms earlier in a college course, they may have been learned out of context rather than being applied to a clinical research article. Along with the language used in research reports, conventions in form (**Table 1**) allow one to find and follow the methodological steps of a study. By understanding where to find the choice of variables, the sampling frame, and the steps of the study, one can better judge its completeness, validity, and relative contribution to research evidence. **Fig. 1** demonstrates how terms fit together and are logically linked to answering questions that provide observable feedback in the form of research outcomes. Each of the building blocks in the article leads to the next step (connected by their function described in oval links).

DEFINITION OF VARIABLES

The term *variable* is drawn from the word *vary,* meaning change, and is used to describe the factors in research. The first rule of thumb for a study variable is that it must be able to have different values or change in the research situation. Factors that do not change in a given study are not variables; they are constants and are sometimes used to exert control. The fact that the same factor might be a variable in one study but a constant or control in another can be confusing if one does not take into consideration the

Table 1
Typical elements of a research report

Section	What it Includes	What it Answers
Introduction	Problem statement Purpose Specific aims Hypotheses/questions Rationale and justification	Why?
Background	Significance Relevant literature Theoretical framework Empirical context of the research Variables selected for study and their definitions Niche the study fills	Why? Why now?
Methods	Design Methods of selecting participants ○ Source ○ Sampling method ○ Eligibility (inclusion and exclusion criteria) Consent procedures How sample size was determined Study procedures Randomization procedures for experiments Methods of measurement ○ Variables and instruments to measure each ○ Reliability and validity of measures ○ Methods to enhance measurement quality Statistical methods ○ Statistical analyses to answer each question or hypothesis ○ Subgroup or adjusted analyses methods ○ Statistical software used	How?
Results	Number and characteristics of sample, subgroups Respondents and nonrespondents Timeline and flow of subjects through study Results addressing each research question or hypothesis Data representing important findings in tables and figures	What?
Discussion	Brief summary of most important findings in context ○ Compared with results of previous studies ○ Related to theoretical framework Discussion of strengths and weaknesses Conclusions and clinical/practice implications Need for further study or questioning	So what?

Adapted from Meininger JC. Mapping out a publishable research report. Presented at the preconference workshop Perish-Proof Publication for Researchers at the Southern Nursing Research Society's 22nd Annual Research Conference. Baltimore, February 11, 2009; with permission.

problem being studied and the question being asked. For example, age might be a variable in a study of preoperative anxiety in elementary school age children; however, if preoperative anxiety was tested only in a group of children on their sixth birthday, age would not be a variable but would be a constant used to control for extraneous effects of age on outcomes. In clinical research we are often most interested in factors that bring about or are associated with a change. These factors are at the very heart of clinical observation; therefore, nurses are usually aware of their variability.

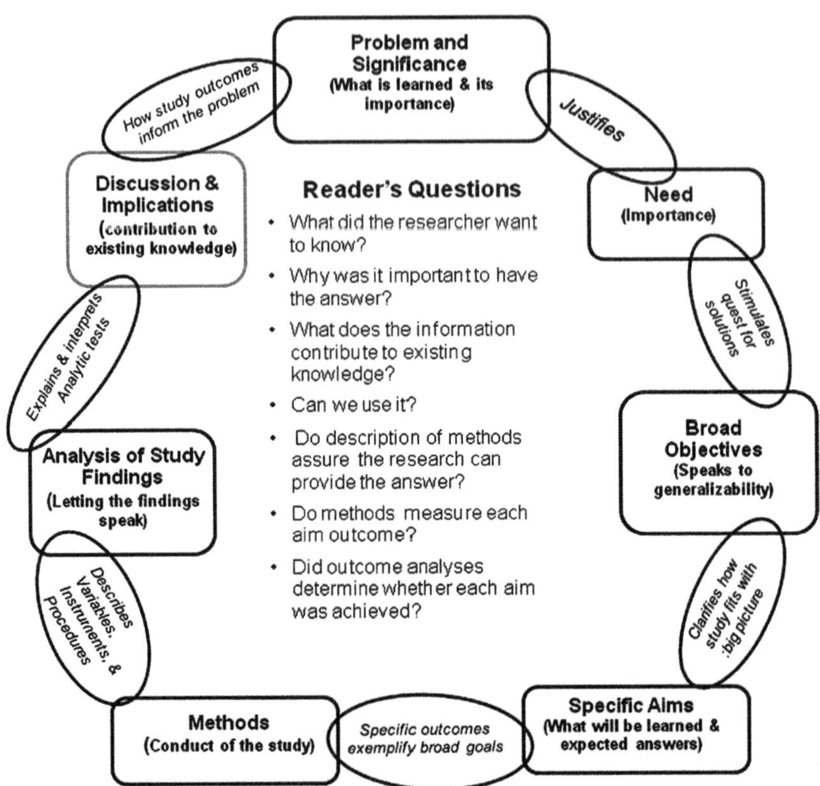

Fig. 1. Chain of logical expectations in reading quantitative research.

INDEPENDENT VERSUS DEPENDENT VARIABLES

Researchers make logical inferences or reasoned expectations about relationships from in-depth knowledge about a topic, observations of behavior, or preliminary studies. In an experimental study, one factor, the independent variable, is manipulated or maneuvered in a way to see its effect on other variables. The variable that shows change is dependent upon the manipulation of the independent variable (which is one way to remember which is which). The independent variable, under the researcher's control and manipulation, does not vary with changes in the dependent variables; rather, it leads to changes in the dependent variable. Independent variables are also called treatment, predictor, grouping, or causal variables, depending on the specific design used. Dependent variables are referred to as outcome variables.

In a study of associations between variables, in which no one is manipulating anything, the researcher may think that one variable might influence another. The term *independent variable* does not fit; therefore, the term *attribute variable* is sometimes used. Examples of attribute variables are found in studies in which one variable, such as age, health status, or acculturation, is studied but not actively manipulated by the researcher and is examined for how it affects a second variable, such as eating habits. Another term, *categorical variable*, is used to describe variables that describe a group or classification of factors that do not have a numerical or hierarchical value, such as gender, ethnicity, religion, or hospital unit, but can be used to group people or things.

IMPORTANCE OF RELATED LITERATURE IN RESEARCH REPORTS

The inclusion of a literature review is not intended to simply inform and orient the reader to the problem under study. Its more essential purpose is to clarify the significance or importance of the study problem and justify the need for the reported research. It puts the reported study into the global perspective of scientific scrutiny with other similar work and sets the scene for discussion of its findings in light of existing knowledge. It provides the context for variable selection and definition by stating what others have found for relationships or differences regarding variables, and how the variables are typically defined in the existing literature. In many studies, the review of literature also provides the theoretical framework or underpinnings for the research, allowing the findings to ultimately be generalized and support, extend, or lead to questioning of theories.

DEFINITION OF A SPECIFIC AIM

The term *specific aim* is sometimes unfamiliar to clinicians who have studied research in college. The term is often neglected in research course work and even in thesis and dissertation supervision, where the focus and vocabulary follows a traditional statement of the problem, purpose, research questions, or hypotheses. Nevertheless, the term is used widely in the research literature, research presentations, and clinical research grant applications. It is actually an action-oriented way of describing outcomes in more detail and is closely linked to the more familiar problem, purpose, or research question. Each element is linked in the following way:

The study problem is usually written as a broad question or proposition addressed by the study (eg, "To what extent does a person's preoperative anxiety state influence their postoperative pain severity?").

The study purpose is stated by examining the proposition in a specific situation (eg, to determine the influence of the preoperative state anxiety on postoperative pain ratings of surgical patients).

Specific aims are outcomes that indicate achievement of the problem and purpose that occur by answering the research questions or testing the study hypotheses. Research reports of quantitative research proposals usually show that the study purpose has been achieved through tests of hypotheses, analyses of cost and benefits, and clear descriptions of previously unknown phenomena (eg, to determine among adolescent males, associations between Amsterdam Anxiety and Information Scale ratings the night before surgery with Visual Analogue Scale pain ratings on the first postoperative day).

RESEARCH QUESTIONS VERSUS HYPOTHESES IN QUANTITATIVE STUDIES

Answerable research questions and testable hypotheses flow directly from specific aims. An aim to describe the measurable characteristics of a group (eg, the average height and weight of preschool children) without drawing an inference or speculating relationships will produce a research question (eg, "What is the mean height and weight of preschool children admitted for tonsillectomy?"). If inferences are to be made and tested quantitatively (eg, relationships between weight and postoperative emergence from anesthesia of preschool children), a research hypotheses is stated (eg, "There is an inverse relationship between body weight and anesthesia emergence time following fentanyl or alfentanil administration."). Without going into elaborate detail, the reader should understand that all hypothesis tests start statistically with the premise of the null hypothesis. In the previously described study, the hypothesis to be statistically tested is "there is no relationship between weight and anesthesia emergence time following fentanyl or alfentanil administration." That is the assumption that there is no difference or relationship. Hypotheses are then tested statistically to determine whether differences or associations found in the study outcomes occurred by chance alone (shown by the *P* for probability value), sometimes called the "level of significance," which is usually set at less than .05. The lower the *P* value, the lower the likelihood that a significant finding happened by chance. For readability and clinical sense, the hypothesis is stated in a research article or proposal as a logical expectation of the outcome, called a "research hypothesis." In the case just mentioned, there is both pharmacologic and physiologic rationale to expect an inverse relationship between weight and the time to emergence from anesthesia.

DESIGNS AS THE BLUEPRINT OF A STUDY

There are dozens of research designs for quantitative research, categorized by the type of data, the timing or frequency of observations, and the number and type of comparative groups and controls. There are elements of research designs beyond the randomization, sampling frames, setting, and control of variables described earlier that form the structure and limitations of a quantitative study. Each of these designs was developed to control the possibility of alternate explanations for relationships or differences found in the study results, or to provide controls for variables extraneous to the study question. How strong or weak a design is to answer a research question depends on how carefully alternate explanations can be ruled out. A few of the designs commonly seen in perioperative literature are described herein.

Cross-sectional studies are those in which data are collected at a single point in time in an effort to explain trends that are characteristics of a population. Because they require less time and expense than longitudinal studies without danger of drop-outs, they are attractive and practical for clinical studies; however, there is a basic weakness in this design because it fails to control for or provide information about relational factors. An example is seen when a one-time test of older adults is used to examine relationships between preoperative knowledge and anxiety level at the time of anesthesia induction. Associations, differences, or characteristics may have many alternate explanations. Major concerns about making inferences about attitudes, behaviors, and developmental characteristics using cross-sectional data include the lack of environmental, experiential, or historical information. To draw accurate clinical inferences from cross-sectional studies, they must be followed by research with longitudinal designs.[11]

Longitudinal designs, repeated measures, or pretest-posttest designs are found in studies with data collected at two or more points in time. Longitudinal studies can be more difficult to conduct in a clinical acute care setting because they require longer participation, follow-up during stays or after discharge from the unit, and consistency of measurement over time. On the other hand, repeated measures designs are particularly suited to studies of physiologic variables being carefully monitored by observation or recorded on clinical devices. Data from repeated measures can be used to record two or more variables over time so that time becomes a point of comparison (eg, to examine associations between blood glucose and core temperature each hour after hypothermic cardiac surgery). Continuous monitoring can also allow repeated measures to be used to measure associations between variables that occur with specific events (eg, to determine if blood glucose levels and core temperatures differ before, during, and after severe shivering). Events such as ambulation, deep cough, or a change of head elevation can be programmed as independent variables in repeated measures to compare the change in dependent variables before, during, and after the event. Pretest-posttest designs are often used to test the effectiveness of an intervention, such as preoperative relaxation training, by measuring the dependent variable (eg, the ability to consciously lower pulse rate) before and after the intervention. This seemingly straight-forward approach, with its directly observable dependent variables, is still open to influence of other extraneous factors. These factors include learning and experience of repeating the measure or simply the passage of time that could possibly influence the second test. Is there something about the persons being tested that influences the outcomes? Some of these factors can be modified by adding a control group whereby one examines whether repeated measurements influence changes in a group without the intervention; however, such designs still might not address whether the people in these groups were initially different in a way that affected the outcome. Each of these weaknesses requires some specific design strategy. Using more than one group to test the intervention, randomizing the assignment of members to each group, and using a control group to simply measure the changes that occur as a function of time are ways to help minimize alternate explanations of outcomes. Some repeated measures studies are suited to having patients serve as their own controls. An example of this approach is seen in a study in which breathing volumes are compared in the same patient without an intervention, after a session of incentive spirometry, and after a treatment of intermittent positive pressure breathing. To avoid bias caused by doing a particular intervention first, the sequence of approaches is randomly varied among all the patients in the study. It is easy to see how clinical studies are full of possible other explanations in the perioperative setting. Variations in dosages and response happen even if the same drugs or anesthetics are given to patients.

INSTRUMENTS AND MEASUREMENT METHODS

Quantitative grant proposals and research articles typically include instruments in their description to help operationalize the variables under study. Operationalizing a variable means describing it in the most objectively measurable, quantifiable, consistent, and valid way possible. Instruments can be data collection structures, scientific devices, biochemical assays, or observational records. Several considerations about instruments in research reports should cause the reader to take note: (1) the validity (legitimacy) or accuracy of the measurement to represent the factor being studied; (2) the precision and sensitivity of the measurement to detect the factor being studied; (3) the chronological availability of the instrument to collect data at the most relevant time; (4) the conditions and reliability or consistency of measurements across the time, conditions, or subjects; and (5) the form of data produced. Both written and physiologic instruments should meet criteria for validity and reliability, and this information should appear for every instrument in the study. Not all variables can be measured directly, particularly those that are reflecting abstract concepts, perceptions, and symptoms. These variables are measured indirectly by questionnaires or checklists and require psychometric refinement to validly represent a particular characteristic. Pen and pencil questionnaires, perceptual scales, attitude surveys, symptom ratings, visual analogue scales, and trait inventories are used widely in perioperative research. Instruments used to measure physiologic variables also require justification for why they are reliable across users and valid in measurement. Medical devices and laboratory assays can have precision without being accurate or valid measurements for the variables under study. For example, serum catecholamines are sometimes used as indicators of anxiety in research. Although these substances may be measured directly and objectively in blood using sophisticated laboratory equipment, they are not direct measures of anxiety alone. Catecholamine levels can be elevated by factors other than anxiety, specifically pain, medications, and circadian variation; therefore, the researcher must justify this choice as a measure and control for competing factors in the design. Descriptions of all study instruments should include the time and method of administration, reliability, validity, and scoring scheme. For scientific devices, descriptions should provide information on the calibration, accuracy, precision, range, and reliability. Specialized devices and laboratory instruments may have specific qualities, such as collection conditions, temperature, and linearity requirements. If variables require laboratory tests or special assays, the collection and storage conditions, reagents or agents, and controls should be provided.

SUFFICIENCY OF STUDY SAMPLES

Studies are rarely conducted on an entire population. Even large epidemiologic studies are done on a smaller, more manageable sample of a larger population. In research, the population is defined by the researcher as all persons, events, or elements having characteristics targeted by a study. Once the population is defined, the researcher must justify and describe how the sample was chosen and provide evidence that it was of sufficient size and representation to support study inferences about the population. Convenience samples are those that are readily available and are the most common in clinical nursing studies; however, it is clear that the easiest persons to enroll in a study might not be the most representative of a population. Convenience samples drawn from hospitals where patients are better educated, healthier, ethnically homogeneous, and younger may yield different results from those with more diversity. Subjects can self-select themselves to participate or not enroll in advertised studies. When the limitations of convenience samples are addressed in research reports, researchers should describe how the limitations affect interpretation of the findings. In studies that include randomized samples, the randomization procedures should be described. Was a random number table used to assign participants before any were selected? Randomization can be as simple as drawing numbers from a hat but may also involve other decisions that affect whether all members of a population have an equal chance of being chosen. Were the numbers returned to the hat to ensure that the number in the hat remained the same for each draw? Were special randomization steps used with treatment and control group assignment to ensure that they ended up with the same number in each group?

SUFFICIENCY OF STUDY POWER: EFFECT SIZE

Achieving a representative sample of a population would logically be more complete when a large sample is gathered; however, large samples are not always possible or even desirable if the researcher is sure there are enough members in the study to detect the effect being studied. The effect size or strength of action of some factors may be so powerful (eg, a postoperative medication to reverse a paralytic drug) that the effect can be seen in everyone. The larger the effect, the easier it will be to demonstrate; however, most clinical effects or study outcomes are not that large, and we must rely on calculations to give us some indication that we have a sample large enough to show the effect if it exists. The ability to detect or be sensitive to a real effect, if it exists, is referred to as a study's power. In planning the sample size needed to deliver sufficient power to detect effects, judgment, pilot work, and knowledge of the researcher come into play. To calculate an appropriate sample size, one considers (1) an expected numerical effect size drawn from pilot work or previous studies; (2) the selected level of significance, conventionally set at .05; and (3) a power goal of 80%, usually considered to be sufficient. The researcher's discussion of effect size and power analysis helps to establish the sensitivity of the study and gives the reader more confidence that study outcomes are not the result of an insufficient sample. Such an example is seen in an excerpt from a report on age-related thermoregulatory differences in a warm operating room environment, "The sample size and power calculations revealed that 30 patients (15 in each group) would be necessary to show a 0.5°C difference in core temperature between the two age groups with a power of 80% and a Type I error protection of 0.05."[12]

DESCRIPTIONS OF PROCEDURES

Because the procedures used in a study are often given only a brief description in a research report, it is difficult to see the procedures linked with the study design or the procedures involved with a particular intervention. Many do not meet the criterion of providing sufficient detail so that someone else could replicate the study. Details as to when randomization took place, who enrolled participants, and who assigned them to groups helps the reader to assess for bias in selection. For studies that involve an educational intervention, the "black box" of what objectives, approaches, materials, and instructional strategies were used is as important as the details of a drug or treatment. Procedures for ensuring responsible conduct of the research study require acknowledgement in the study, ranging from the approval of the hospital or agency's institutional review board to the method of securing informed consent of participants. Most professional journals are now requiring this information as a part of all published research involving human subjects.

DATA ANALYSIS LINKS WITH STUDY RESULTS

In quantitative research reports, data analysis is conducted to describe and test relationships between variables. Space limitations often lead researchers to describe the analytic procedures along with the results and can leave the reader wondering what analyses were done to test for specified relationships or differences. The notion of a roadmap becomes useful in helping readers as follows: (1) look at each specific aim, research question, or hypothesis; (2) try to find the variable and unit of measurement for each question or test; and (3) seek the specific statistical test used to test each relationship. Sometimes the reader will find a generalized statement such as, "Differences in continuous variables were determined using analysis of variance, and associations between categorical variables were assessed using χ^2 or Fisher's exact tests."[13] Although the information is there, the reader will have to determine which variables were continuous, which were categorical, and which tests were used for which categorical variables. Studies that are more explicit in connecting the questions to the statistical procedures are easier to read. It is particularly helpful when the report tells how complex or continuous data are captured and analyzed. In the following example taken from a study of the effects of two warming devices on body heat content and core temperature, an entire section of the article explains the conversion of oxygen consumption to equivalent metabolic heat production and careful calculation of body heat content. There is no doubt about how these data were analyzed because the section explicitly tells how data were condensed and tested.[14]

> *Values during the control periods were first averaged within each volunteer and then averaged among the volunteers. Potential confounding factors were compared with paired t tests and are expressed as mean ± SD. The rate at which core temperature increased was evaluated by regression from 60 to 120 elapsed minutes (the linear portion of the curve). Results comparing temperature and heat content between the two treatments are expressed as mean with 95% confidence interval and displayed in the figures.*

Results in research reports contain findings or the bare facts revealed by the data analysis. Unfortunately, this section may seem like dry reading to those who want answers to the questions posed at the article's beginning. This section may begin with some of the demographic findings and descriptive statistics for study variables. Ideally, the statistical findings on each of the study questions or hypothesis are presented in the order they were stated in the beginning of the article. If you have followed the roadmap suggested earlier in your reading of the specific aims, questions or hypotheses, and measurements, it will be easier to search for the results that provide the answers. Take advantage of any graphs or tables the author provides. Graphs often show visual variations that make the numerical findings more meaningful. Avoid skipping over the results so you are sure that the discussion accurately represents the actual findings.

THE DISCUSSION: INTERPRETING THE RESULTS

The discussion section interprets the results for a scientific or clinical reader, offering explanatory details for known relationships and speculations for those that cannot be verified. It should be clear in this discussion whether any hypothesized relationships were supported, or if there were unexpected findings. Weaknesses in design or sampling that could explain these findings should be included. The earlier review of relevant literature provides a backdrop against which the present findings are discussed. If a theoretical framework was used, the discussion should point out if the framework was supported or refuted by the findings, or if the results were equivocal. Study results should be sized up as to their contribution to existing research and knowledge. Do the findings conflict or are they congruent with existing research? Do the findings clearly suggest implications for future research as new research? Do the findings contribute to the scientific body of knowledge beyond that of the present study?

THE CONCLUSION: THE AUTHORS AND THE READERS

In research articles, the term *conclusion* means more than the end of the article. Research articles vary in whether they include a section or simply a paragraph with conclusions about the study. Conclusions may be just one sentence such as, "In conclusion, upper body forced-air warming is more effective than the heating pad for maintaining body temperature intraoperatively."[15] Alternatively, they may include a summary of deductions that suggest future research. Comments about implications for clinical practice are often included in this section or in the discussion. It is the last opportunity for the researcher to make a point about what he or she concluded from the study and to generalize about its importance to a wider scientific community. Ask yourself at the point of reading conclusions, "Do the study findings and interpretation offer me something I can use?"

Table 2
Reading roadmap for quantitative research

What Do You Want to Find?	Where Can You Find It?	How Can You Evaluate this Study Element?
What were the researchers trying to find out and why?	Problem, purpose Specific aims Hypotheses/questions Background and significance Review of related literature	Do problem, purpose, specific aims "hang together?" Was existing knowledge reviewed? Was it clear how the study would contribute to knowledge? Is literature from both sides of an issue reviewed? Were you convinced of the need for the study?
Who and how many did they study?	Methodology section Sample description Setting	Is diversity and regional location of the sample described? Are exclusions justified? Are limitations in sample described?
Did they justify the number they selected?	Sampling strategy Effect size and power analysis Data analysis	Was sampling strategy and power analysis described? Was effect size estimate from pilot or prior study? Were power analysis findings linked to statistical tests?
How did they select a sample?	Sampling strategy Study procedures Informed consent	Was the study randomized in any way? If not randomized, was a systematic inclusion plan described? Were there measures to ensure representation? Are informed consent procedures described?
Do you know of a similar population or setting?	Sample description Setting	From what you know about similar populations and settings, do the plans and controls seem reasonable?
What data did they gather and did it measure the desired variables?	Methodology section Variables/instruments	Are the selection of measuring devices, validity, and reliability well justified? Were extraneous variables controlled for?
Did they describe what statistics they used in the data analyses and whether they were used to describe, compare, or correlate variables?	Methodology section Data analysis Results Tabled values	Were data analyses generalized and nonspecific? Were analytic procedures related to specific aims? Were actual statistics provided or only *P* values?
What did they find out and what did they conclude?	Results Discussion/conclusion	Were conclusions congruent with findings or overstated? Were findings discussed in light of aims or existing knowledge?
Do the study findings and conclusions make sense and concur with your own experience or understanding?	Results Discussion/conclusion	From your own expertise do conclusions seem reasonable? Are there alternate reasons that might account for findings?

THE "TAKE-HOME" MESSAGE FROM THE ARTICLE

Perioperative nurses who become comfortable reading clinical research find that it contributes to their awareness of relationships in practice. Their expertise may make them aware that statistically significant outcomes of studies can often occur with only tiny variations in clinical outcomes and little implication for practice applications, highlighting the difference between statistical and clinical significance. For example, a recent study featured by the editor of a scholarly nursing journal showed a statistically significant difference in hemoglobin level of 14 in one group and 13.6 in another group.[16] Clinical experts recognize that these differences are not clinically significant, and that statistical significance simply means that the tiny outcome did not likely occur by chance alone. Beyond this, nurses are sometimes uncertain how to apply findings or judging when an effective intervention is ready to implement. Reading a research article is more interesting when you have others to discuss your "take-home" understanding. **Table 2** provides a reading roadmap for evaluating quantitative research articles that can help readers find and ask questions from a particular article. Global questions the reader might want to ask appear in the first column, where to locate the answer is listed in the second column, and specific elements related to the question that will require the reader's evaluation of the article are listed in the third column. Areas on the roadmap that seem difficult to understand, such as effect size and power analysis, can be made less formidable by discussions with user-friendly clinical or faculty researchers.

Whether colleagues have a formal journal club to discuss research articles, spend time at chapter meetings of the Association of Operating Room Nurses to discuss an article's application of research, or just chat about such reading over coffee, they assume the important role of evaluating a study's merit. The published study enjoys the benefit of being held up to the light of scientific rigor by some of the most important consumers of research—nurse clinicians in perioperative practice.

REFERENCES

1. Mitchell PH. Research and development in nursing revisited: nursing science as the basis for evidence-based practice. J Adv Nurs 2006;54(5):528–9.
2. American Society of PeriAnesthesia Nurses PONV PDNV Strategic Work Team. ASPAN'S evidence-based clinical practice guideline for the prevention and/or management of PONV/PDNV. J Perianesth Nurs 2006;21(4):230–50.
3. Girard NJ, Girard NJ. Standards, recommended practices, and guidelines. AORN J 2006;83(2):307–8.
4. Good KK, Verble JA, Secrest J, et al. Postoperative hypothermia: the chilling consequences. AORN J 2006;83(5):1054–66 [quiz: 1067–70].
5. Hoss B, Hanson D, Hoss B, et al. Evaluating the evidence: web sites. AORN J 2008;87(1):124–41.
6. Campbell DT, Stanley JC. Experimental and quasi-experimental designs for research. Chicago: Rand McNally; 1963.
7. Sawilowsky SS. ANCOVA and quasi-experimental design: the legacy of Campbell and Stanley. In: Sawilowsky SS, editor. Real data analysis. Charlotte (NC): Information Age Publishing; 2007. p. 213–40.
8. Harris AD, Bradham DD, Baumgarten M, et al. The use and interpretation of quasi-experimental studies in infectious diseases. Clin Infect Dis 2004;38(11): 1586–91.
9. Yeh ML, Yang HJ, Chen HH, et al. Using a patient-controlled analgesia multimedia intervention for improving analgesia quality. J Clin Nurs 2007;16(11):2039–46.

10. Polit DF, Beck CT. Nursing research: generating and assessing evidence for nursing practice. 8th edition. Philadelphia: Lippincott, Williams & Wilkins; 2008.
11. Kraemer HC, Yesavage JA, Taylor JL, et al. How can we learn about developmental processes from cross-sectional studies, or can we? Am J Psychiatry 2000;157(2):163–71.
12. El-Gamal N, El-Kassabany N, Frank SM, et al. Age-related thermoregulatory differences in a warm operating room environment (approximately 26 degrees C). Anesth Analg 2000;90(3):694–8.
13. Ng SF, Oo CS, Loh KH, et al. A comparative study of three warming interventions to determine the most effective in maintaining perioperative normothermia. Anesth Analg 2003;96(1):171–6 [table of contents].
14. Taguchi A, Ratnaraj J, Kabon B, et al. Effects of a circulating-water garment and forced-air warming on body heat content and core temperature. Anesthesiology 2004;100(5):1058–64.
15. Leung KK, Lai A, Wu A. A randomised controlled trial of the electric heating pad vs forced-air warming for preventing hypothermia during laparotomy. Anaesthesia 2007;62(6):605–8.
16. Gennaro S. Sign of significance. J Nurs Scholarsh 2008;40(2):99–100.

Viewing the Rich, Diverse Landscape of Qualitative Research

Cheryl Tatano Beck, DNSc, CNM, FAAN

KEYWORDS

- Qualitative research • Phenomenology • Grounded theory
- Meta-synthesis • Narrative analysis • Ethnography

The power of qualitative research is gripping. It provides nurses with a privileged glimpse in the world of their patients, frightening and horrifying as it is at times. Qualitative research allows nurses and other health care providers an opportunity to walk a mile in the shoes of their patients so they can better design interventions to help improve the quality of their patients' lives. Qualitative research helps make the invisible visible. For example, in the author's qualitative study of mothers' anniversaries of their traumatic childbirth experiences[1] an invisible phenomenon was discovered. The celebration each year of the child's birthday was in fact, for these women who suffered birth trauma, a tormented day where family, friends, and clinicians failed to rescue them. As one mother painfully shared, "Every birthday is no longer the celebration of the child, but is really an anniversary for the rape."[1] In Beck's qualitative studies on birth trauma and its resulting posttraumatic stress disorder because of childbirth,[2,3] the most frequent image women used to describe their traumatic births was that it was like being raped on the delivery table, with everyone watching and no one offering to help.

In this article, six of the most common qualitative research designs are discussed: phenomenology, grounded theory, ethnography, historical research, narrative analysis, and meta-synthesis. Some of these research designs are illustrated by concrete examples from the author's research program on postpartum mood and anxiety disorders, and others are examples from published studies in perioperative nursing. The article ends with a discussion of criteria to assess the rigor of qualitative research.

Qualitative research stems from the naturalistic paradigm. This paradigm provides the blueprint for different methods for conducting nursing research that are dramatically in contrast to those of the positivistic paradigm, which guides quantitative research. For the discipline of nursing, which deals with human complexity, both traditional quantitative research methods and the exciting qualitative research methods are needed for the discovery of knowledge to improve nursing care and the quality of life of our patients.

School of Nursing, University of Connecticut, 231 Glenbrook Road, Storrs, CT 06269-2026, USA
E-mail address: cheryl.beck@uconn.edu

Perioperative Nursing Clinics 4 (2009) 217–229
doi:10.1016/j.cpen.2009.05.006 periopnursing.theclinics.com
1556-7931/09/$ – see front matter

In the naturalistic paradigm an assumption is that reality is not fixed, but instead is multiple. Reality is subjective and discovered from persons participating in research. As a result, there are multiple interpretations of reality. Also in the naturalistic paradigm, the results of a study are created by the interaction between the researcher and the participants. Knowledge is best discovered when the distance between the researcher and participants is minimized.[4] Unlike in quantitative research, where objectivity is the gold standard, the subjective nature of qualitative inquiry is acknowledged and accepted. These assumptions of the naturalistic paradigm have major implications for how qualitative research is designed and conducted. Qualitative research uses an inductive process and flexible, emergent designs, deriving generalizations from specific experiences. Emphasis is on the holistic understanding of complex human experience.

Just as quantitative research has different research designs to choose from, depending upon the research question being investigated, so does qualitative research. Qualitative research is viewed by some individuals as a soft science, as a second-class citizen to quantitative research. Part of the reason for this erroneous perception is the lack of knowledge and understanding of the rigorous, intricate research methods in the naturalistic paradigm. A frequent erroneous belief is that there is just one general qualitative research design available to researchers: that being, to interview participants and look for themes. Nothing can be further from the truth. Consider the differing approaches in each of the following six types of qualitative designs.

PHENOMENOLOGY

Research Design

Phenomenology is both a philosophy and a research method. The goal of the phenomenologic method is to describe human experience as it is lived without theories about the cause of the experience.[5] It is the study of essences and is derived from the Greek word "phenomenon," which means to show itself. The method is rooted in a philosophic tradition developed by Husserl[6] and Heidegger.[7] Heightened awareness of the researcher's consciousness, presuppositions, and biases in advance regarding the phenomenon under study is critical. What is done with this heightened awareness differentiates the two types of phenomenology, descriptive and interpretive, and how data are collected and analyzed.

The origin of descriptive phenomenology is from the philosophy of Husserl,[6] who is called "the father of phenomenology." Husserl was a mathematican before becoming a philosopher and used the term "bracketing" to describe the process of reduction, whereby researchers identify their own presuppositions about the phenomenon being studied and bring them into their consciousness so they can deliberately set them aside and reduce their bias of the data. Phenomenologic researchers do not want to view the phenomenon under study though their lens of preconceived notions. Fink, as cited by Merleau-Ponty, stated that in order for researchers to describe lived experience, they must be "astonished before the world."[8] Merleau-Ponty[8] goes on to argue, however, that complete reduction, which Husserl called for, can never be fully accomplished.

This debate over complete reduction led to the development of interpretive phenomenology. Heidegger was Husserl's student and moved away from his professor's philosophic stance. Heidegger[7] believed one must go beyond description to interpreting human experience. What researchers bring into their consciousness about the phenomenon being studied is not set aside or bracketed. Because Heidegger strongly believed that researchers are always being-in-the-world, their beliefs and experiences are an important part of the research process. Researchers' raised consciousness levels are brought to the table in interpretive phenomenology. In interpretive phenomenology, shared experiences of the researcher's and participant's of being-in-the-world is the goal.

Research Question

A typical research question for a phenomenologic study would be stated as: What is the essence of a phenomenon as experienced by a group of people and what does this experience mean to them? In the author's descriptive phenomenologic study of the experience of postpartum depression, her research question was: What is the essence of women's experiences of postpartum depression?[9]

Sample

Purposive sampling is used in phenomenology. Participants are purposely invited to be included in the sample because they have experienced the phenomenon being studied. Sample size is usually much smaller than that needed for a quantitative study. Typical sample size for a phenomenologic study is 12 or fewer individuals.[10] The meaningfulness and insights generated from qualitative data have more to do with the information richness of the participants' descriptions than with sample size.[11] Phenomenologists recruit new participants until they reach what is called "data saturation." This occurs when no new themes emerge and there is repetition of the responses from participants. In Beck's[9] phenomenologic study her purposive sample consisted of seven mothers who were suffering from postpartum depression. In Beck's study, 11 themes emerged that described the essence of mothers' experiences of postpartum depression. After five interviews Beck did not identify any additional, new themes. Data replicated and verified the earlier themes. Beck interviewed two more mothers just to make sure she had reached data saturation.

Data Collection

In-depth interviews are the primary source of data collection in phenomenologic studies. The interviews are usually started off with a broad request asking the participants to describe their experience of the phenomenon being studied. In Beck's[9] study the seven women were each asked to respond to the following statement: "Please describe a situation in which you experienced postpartum depression. Share all the thoughts, perceptions, and feelings you can recall until you have no more to say about the situation."[9] The interview format usually remains invariant during the whole process of data collection in phenomenology.

Data Analysis

Colaizzi,[12] Giorgi,[13] and Van Kaam's[14] methods are examples of approaches to data analysis in descriptive phenomenology frequently used by nurse researchers. A comparison of the steps involved in these three methods can be found in Beck's[15] article on reliability and validity issues in phenomenologic research. No matter what method is chosen, phenomenologists search for common patterns or themes that together describe the essence of the phenomenon under study.

Colaizzi's[12] method is described here as an example of phenomenologic data analysis. Once the interviews have been transcribed, Colaizzi calls for extracting significant statements from each transcription. Significant statements are phrases, sentences, and paragraphs that the participants have said that are specific to the phenomenon under study. These significant statements are then categorized into clusters of themes. These themes are then checked back with the original transcripts to validate them. Next, an exhaustive description of the phenomenon under study is written. In this exhaustive description, all the findings to date are integrated into as complete a description of the essence of the experience as possible. The final step consists of the researcher going back to the participants to validate the results.

Colaizzi's[12] method was used in Beck's[9] descriptive phenomenologic study of postpartum depression. Analysis of the transcripts of the in-depth interviews yielded 11 themes. Some examples of these themes included "Theme 2: Contemplating death provided a glimmer of hope to the end of their living nightmare," "Theme 4: Haunted by the fear that any normalcy in their lives was irretrievable, the mothers grieved for their loss of self," and "Theme 8: Mothers envisioned themselves as robots stripped of all positive feelings, just going through the motions."[9]

Examples of commonly used interpretive phenomenologic methods by nurse researchers include Van Manen[16] and Benner.[17]

GROUNDED THEORY

Research Design

Grounded theory is an inductive qualitative research method created by two sociologists, Glaser and Strauss.[18] The goal of grounded theory is to discover the basic social psychologic problem/central concern in a substantive area, such as postpartum depression, and to identify the process used to resolve this central concern. The grounded theorist generates a theory around what Glaser and Strauss called a "core category." A core category accounts for most of the pattern of behavior that is relevant or problematic for persons in a substantive area. The other categories in a grounded theory are related to the core category that has as its primary function the integrating of the theory. One type of core category that is often reported in nursing research studies is a basic social process, which evolves over time and has at last two clear stages. Stages have a dimension of time. The stages have a perceivable start and end.

Research Question

An example of a grounded theory research question comes from Beck's[19] grounded theory study of postpartum depression entitled "Teetering on the Edge." The research questions investigated were: What is the specific social psychologic problem women experience in postpartum depression? What social psychologic process is used to resolve this fundamental problem?

Sample

Theoretic sampling is used in grounded theory. In this type of sampling, subsequent recruitment of participants is based on the theory developing from previous participants' data. Selection of sample members is based on ensuring adequate representation of the theoretical categories as they develop.

Data Collection and Data Analysis

A basic feature of grounded theory is simultaneous data collection and data analysis. Because of this, grounded theory is often called the "constant comparative method." This procedure is used to generate conceptual categories and their properties and integrate them into a substantive theory grounded in the data.

In phenomenology, in-depth interviewing is the primary method used to collect data. More sources of data are open to grounded theorists to use in addition to interviews, such as participant observation and review of documents. The interviewing technique in grounded theory is different than the approach used in phenomenology. As the concepts are generated and linked together in the grounded theory approach, the interviewing technique changes. At the start of the study, the interviews are unstructured and participants are asked to describe their experiences. As the theory develops, the questions become much more focused and specific. The interview questions are now related to categories in the developing grounded theory. Interviews tend to get shorter as the grounded theory develops because the questions are more specific and can be answered more quickly.

Coding is used to analyze data in grounded theory.[20] Codes are just labels given to data that capture what is going on. There are two main coding types: (*i*) substantive codes that are used to conceptualize the substance of the topic being studied and (*ii*) theoretic codes that link substantive codes together to generate a grounded theory. Theoretic codes allow grounded theory to have an in-depth explanatory power because they increase the abstract meaning of the relationships among categories.[21] Originally, Glaser[22] provided grounded theorists with 18 families of theoretic codes to help them to determine how substantive codes relate to each other conceptually. Examples of these coding families include strategy, process, and critical junctures. Recently, Glaser[21] expanded his initial 18 families of theoretic codes to an endless list of possibilities from a wide array of disciplines. One example of his new theoretic coding is amplifying causal looping from the discipline of economics.

Fig. 1 presents the four-stage process of teetering on the edge[19] to help illustrate both types of coding and what the outcome of a grounded theory study looks like. Loss of control of their emotions and thought processes was the basic problem women experienced in postpartum depression. They resolved this central problem through the four stages listed in **Fig. 1**. Under each of the four stages are three arrows to boxes. In these boxes are substantive codes, such as enveloping fogginess and alarming unrealness. At the bottom of the figure under each stage are examples of theoretic codes that link one stage to another, such as conditions, consequences, and strategies.

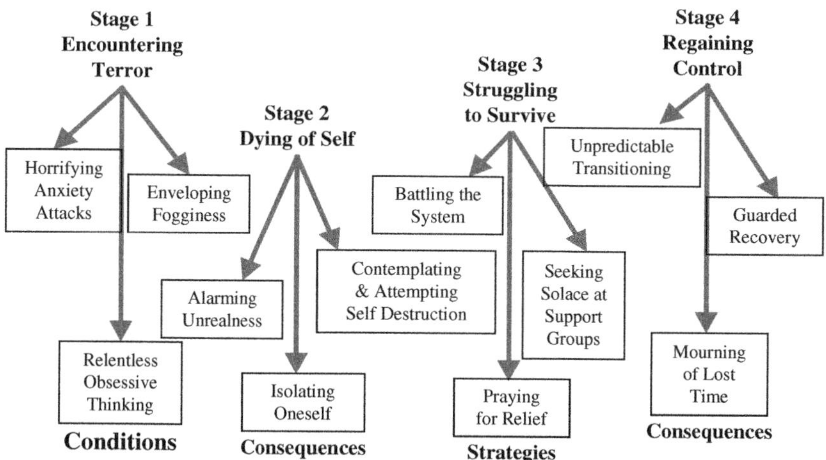

Fig. 1. Four-stage process of teetering on the edge. (*From* Beck CT. Teetering on the edge: a substantive theory of postpartum depression. Nurs Res 1993;42:43; with permission.)

ETHNOGRAPHY

Research Design

Ethnography is a qualitative research approach that comes from the discipline of anthropology. It is concerned with cultural patterns and experiences. The lifeways of cultures or subcultures are examined. Depending on how broad or how narrow the focus of the study is determines whether it is classified as either a macro-ethnography or a micro- (focused) ethnography.

Research Question

Ethnographers investigate research questions that ask, for example, what are the patterns of behavior of persons in a specific culture regarding health and illness?

Sample

Participants in an ethnographic study are often called "informants." Critical to the success of this type of qualitative research are key informants who are well versed in the culture and topic being studied. They provide great insight and valuable information to the researcher.

Data Collection

A crucial step in ethnography is gaining entry into the culture being studied. Extensive field work in the culture is the hallmark of this type of qualitative design. A strategy called "participant observation" may be used. In participant observation the researcher observes the behaviors of persons in a culture while also participating in their activities. This helps ethnographers to immerse themselves in the culture. Extensive field notes are written during data collection.

Data Analysis

The outcomes of analysis of field notes, participant observation, interviews, and documents are patterns or themes in the behavior and thoughts of the informants regarding aspects of their cultural lifeways. There are different approaches to data analysis in ethonography. Spradley's[23] research sequence is one such approach. Spradley's method relies heavily on language as the primary way that cultural meaning is obtained. He calls for four levels of data analysis: domain, taxonomic, componential, and theme analysis. Leininger and McFarland[24] provided another approach in their four-phase ethnonursing data analysis guide. The first phase includes collecting and recording data. The second phase focuses on identifying and categorizing descriptors of the culture. Next, repetitive patterns are discovered. In the fourth phase major themes are abstracted.

Gillespie, Wallis, and Chaboyer[25] conducted an ethnographic study of the culture of the operating theater in Australia. It is considered a mini or focused ethnography, the aim of which was "to explore characteristics of organizational culture of the operating theater and how this culture is communicated and sustained. The field setting was an 8-theater department in a major hospital in Queensland, Australia. Informants included nurses, orderlies, trainee and consultant surgeons and anesthetists."[25] Their fieldwork took place over a 6-week period that included five 6-hour days per week, for a total of 180 hours. Three themes evolved from data analysis that dealt with the primacy of knowledge and competence, social order, and situational control. These themes have implications for nurse retention.

HISTORICAL RESEARCH

Research Design

Historical research is a qualitative approach in which there is the systematic collection, critical assessment, and interpretation of historical data. Historical research examines events, persons, or a particular period in nursing's past. Historians believe that examining nursing's past will help us to better understand contemporary nursing.

Research Questions

Historians investigate questions focusing on causes, effects, and trends in regard to past events that may help us to understand present practices in nursing. Other types of research questions seek to answer questions about a person's life or a specific period in their life.

Sample

In historical research, the sample can consist of various types of historical data, such as interview data, written documents, diaries, letters, pictures, meeting minutes, and so forth. Sometimes the sample may not even include a person if the event or individual the historian is researching is so far in the past that no one from that era is still living.

Data Collection

Data in historical research are categorized as primary or secondary sources. Primary sources are first-hand information or accounts regarding the event or person being studied, while secondary sources are second- or third-hand accounts. Primary sources are the preferred sources of data in an historical study.

Data Analysis

A critical task for historians is evaluating the historical data they have found. This task is twofold. First, the researcher is concerned with external criticism. Here the authenticity of the data is examined. Next is internal criticism, where the historian evaluates the worth of the content of the data. Is the evidence accurate?

Harris and Hunziker-Dean[26] provided an example of an historical study in the perioperative specialty. The title of their study was "Florence Henderson: The art of open-drop ether." This historical study focused on the life, education, work, and publications of one nurse, Florence Henderson, at the turn of the twentieth century. Her work was dedicated to the art of delivering anesthesia. Florence Henderson contributed to developing ether administration techniques and to establishing criteria to assess anesthetized patients. This nurse anesthetist was a pioneer in advocating for the role of nurse specialists in anesthesia. In 1909 at the 12th Annual Convention of the Nurses' Associated Alumnae of the United States, she presented her paper "The Nurse as an Anaesthetist." In 1913 she presented another paper, "Ether Anesthesia," at the Southern Minnesota Medical Association.

NARRATIVE ANALYSIS

Research Design

Narrative analysis is the qualitative research design that focuses on story as the object of the investigation.[27,28] Narratives are ways in which individuals make sense of events in their lives. Reissman views narratives as cultural envelopes into which individuals pour their experiences. What distinguishes narrative analysis from phenomenology and other qualitative research designs is that the participants' stories are kept as wholes and not divided up.

Research Question

An example of research questions for a narrative analysis include: What story does a person have to tell? How do persons make sense of the events in their lives?

Sample

There is no set sample size required for narrative analysis. Some narrative analyses have been published with a sample size of 1, while others have included a sample of 35 participants.

Data Collection and Data Analysis

Interviews and documents are the primary means of collecting data. Just as in phenomenology, where qualitative researchers have a choice of approaches to analyze the data, there are also choices in narratives analysis. Researchers should choose their approach based on the fit with the type of narratives to be analyzed. Three of the more popular structural approaches are those of Gee,[29] Labov and Waletzky,[30] and Burke.[31]

Gee's[29] approach is a linguistic approach to narrative analysis that focuses on changes in pitch, pauses, and other punctuations of speech. The narrative is divided up into lines, stanzas, and strophes. Lines make up stanzas and then stanzas are paired into strophes. To use Gee's structural approach the narrative must have been tape-recorded and transcribed.

Labov and Waletzky's[30] structural approach is composed of six components: the abstract (the summary), orientation (time, place, persons), complicating action (sequence of events), evaluation (significance of the action), resolution (result, what happened at the end), and coda (perspective returned to the present).

Burke's[31] structural approach for narrative analysis is called "dramatistic pentad." There are five key elements of a story according to Burke: act (what took place), scene (backdrop of the act), agent (individual who performed the act), agency (means or instruments the agent used), and purpose (the why of the act). His pentad of terms are not meant to be analyzed as individual components but instead as ratio of the elements paired together, such as scene is to agent or act is to agency. Each ratio of terms provide the narrative analysts with different ways to view the story. Burke calls the pairing of terms "terministic screens," an approach for helping to open up an analyst's perspective. His pairing of terms helps to reveal the imbalances in the pentadic ratios.

To illustrate a concrete example of narrative analysis, Beck's[32] study of birth trauma narratives is described here. The sample included 11 mothers who had experiences a traumatic birth. These women sent their narratives to the researcher via the Internet. Six women were from the United States, three from New Zealand, one from Australia, and one from the United Kingdom. For the analysis of these birth-trauma stories, Burke's[31] dramatistic pentad was chosen. Analysis revealed that the most frequent ratio imbalance or problematic area in the narratives was the ratio of act to agency. What was so traumatic for the women about their childbirth was how actions were done to them by the clinicians. **Table 1** lists the ratio imbalances that occurred in each of the 11 narratives. The glaring absence of caring and communication during their childbirth came out loud and clear, as indicated by the predominance of the imbalance between act and agency.

Table 1
Birth trauma narratives with corresponding ratio imbalances

Participant	Birth Trauma	Ratio	Imbalance
1	On the postpartum unit delivery of a nonliving preterm infant	Scene 1 Scene 2 Scene 3	Scene:Agent Act:Agency Act:Agency
2	Emergency cesarean of a preterm infant due to mother's hemorrhaging; infant to neonatal intensive care unit	Scene 1 Scene 2	Act:Agency Scene:Agent
3	Emergency cesarean due to "baby being stuck"	Scene 1	Act:Agent
4	Hemorrhaging due to vasa previa; emergency cesarean	Scene 1 Scene 2	Act:Agency Act:Agent
5	Multiple insertions for epidural; mother's blood pressure dropped; fetal heart rate dropped, leading to a crisis	Scene 1 Scene 2	Act:Agency Act:Agency
6	Mother sustained nerve damage due to two forceps deliveries of her twins; her left foot and leg paralyzed	Scene 1 Scene 2 Scene 3 Scene 4	Scene:Agent Act:Agency Act:Agency Agent:Act
7	Postpartum hemorrhage after water birth	Scene 1	Scene:Agent
8	Epidural did not work, but labor and delivery (L&D) staff did not believe mother; forceps delivery without pain medication	Scene 1	Act:Agency
9	Mother in active labor, but L&D staff did not believe her; vacuum extraction without any pain medication; mother hemorrhaged	Scene 1 Scene 2	Act:Agency Act:Agency
10	Mother induced against her wishes; first twin delivered vaginally; second twin delivered by cesarean	Scene 1 Scene 2 Scene 3	Act:Agency Act:Agency Act:Agency
11	Mother's pelvis dislocated when nurse yanked bedpan away	Scene 1 Scene 2	Act:Agency Act:Agency

From Beck CT. Pentadic cartography: mapping birth trauma narratives. Qual Health Res 2006;16:459; with permission.

META-SYNTHESIS

Research Design

Meta-synthesis is to qualitative studies as meta-analysis is to quantitative studies. Meta-synthesis is "the bringing together and breaking down of findings, examining them, discovering the essential features and, in some way, combining phenomena into a transformed whole."[33] In a meta-synthesis, findings from qualitative studies on the same topic are translated into each other to come up with something more than the sum of their parts. Sandelowski and Barroso refer to meta-syntheses as "both an interpretive product and to the analytic processes by which the findings of studies are integrated, compared or otherwise put together."[34] With the current emphasis on evidence-based practice and ways to increase the utility of qualitative research results, meta-synthesis is viewed a valuable source of evidence for clinical practice. With the help of meta-syntheses, qualitative research is beginning to secure the place it deserves in evidence-based practice.[35]

Sample

The sample in a meta-synthesis consists of published and unpublished qualitative studies. A researcher sets criteria for which studies will and will not be included in the meta-synthesis.

Data Collection

A thorough review of the literature across disciplines is conducted to locate all the qualitative studies on the topic being examined. Online data bases such as CINAHL, PsycLit, PubMed, and Dissertation Abstracts are reviewed.

Data Analysis

Noblit and Hare's[36] approach for synthesizing qualitative studies is used frequently by nurse researchers. Once the researcher has decided on a phenomenon to study and has located all the qualitative studies relevant to this topic, Noblit and Hare identified three possible ways studies can be related to each other "(1) the accounts are directly comparable as 'reciprocal' translations; (2) the accounts stand in relative opposition to each other and are essentially 'refutational'; or (3) the studies taken together present a 'line of argument' rather than a reciprocal or refutational translation."[36]

The following are Noblit and Hare's steps in their approach to conducting a metasynthesis:

Translating studies into one another. As Noblit and Hare explained, "Translations are especially unique syntheses, because they protect the particular, respect holism, and enable comparison. An adequate translation maintains the central metaphors and/or concepts of each account in their relation to other key metaphors or concepts in that account."[36]

Synthesizing translations. A whole is created that is something more than the individual parts imply.

Expressing the results of the meta-synthesis in written form, plays, artwork, videos, or music.

Beck[37] conducted a meta-synthesis using Noblit and Hare's[36] approach to synthesizing 18 qualitative studies on postpartum depression. This synthesis included six studies in the United States, eight in the United Kingdom, three in Australia, and one in Canada. This meta-synthesis took the form of reciprocal translations because the studies were about similar things. With reciprocal translations, each study was translated into the metaphors of the others and vice versa. These 18 studies involved a total of 309 mothers suffering from postpartum depression. In synthesizing these studies' results, four themes emerged that reflected the primary perspectives involved with postpartum depression: (1) incongruity between expectations and reality of motherhood, (2) spiraling downward, (3) pervasive loss, and (4) making gains.

ASSESSING THE QUALITY OF QUALITATIVE RESEARCH

There are various frameworks to choose from that can be used to critique a qualitative study for its rigor. Sandelowski[38] stressed the need for different criteria in assessing qualitative research than for those used in quantitative research: "We can preserve or kill the spirit of qualitative work; we can soften our notion of rigor to include the playfulness, soulfulness, imagination, and technique we associate with more artistic

Table 2
Assessment of primary and secondary criteria of validity

Criteria	Assessment
Primary criteria	
Credibility	Do the results of the research reflect the experience of participants or the context in a believable way?
Authenticity	Does a representation of the emic perspective exhibit awareness to the subtle differences in the voices of all participants?
Criticalityvc	Does the research process demonstrate evidence of critical appraisal?
Integrity	Does the research reflect recursive and repetitive checks of validity as well as a humble presentation of findings?
Secondary criteria	
Explicitness	Have methodologic decisions, interpretations, and investigator biases been addressed?
Vividness	Have thick and faithful descriptions been portrayed with artfulness and clarity?
Creativity	Have imaginative ways of organizing, presenting, and analyzing data been incorporated?
Thoroughness	Do the findings convincingly address the questions posed through completeness and saturation?
Congruence	Are the process and the findings congruent? Do all the themes fit together? Do findings fit into a context outside the study situation?
Sensitivity	Has the investigation been implemented in ways that are sensitive to the nature of human, cultural, and social contexts?

From Whittemore R, Chase SK, Mandle CL. Validity in qualitative research. Qual Health Res 2001; 11:534; with permission.

endeavors. Or we can further harden it by the uncritical application of rules. The choice is ours; rigor or rigor mortis."[38] The framework most frequently cited for quality criteria for qualitative research is one developed by Lincoln and Guba[39] and then revised by Guba and Lincoln.[40] Their five criteria for assessing the trustworthiness of qualitative research included credibility, dependability, confirmability, transferability, and authenticity. Whittemore and colleagues[41] proposed another framework that was composed of primary and secondary qualitative validity criteria. Their primary criteria address credibility, authenticity, criticality, and integrity. Secondary criteria include explicitness, vividness, creativity, thoroughness, congruence, and sensitivity. **Table 2** lists specific questions that can be used to assess Whittemore and colleagues' criteria.

In conclusion, six qualitative research designs were chosen to describe as an introduction to some of the varied landscape of qualitative research. There are many other types of qualitative landscapes available to nurse researchers, such as participatory action research and discourse analysis, to name a couple. For clinicians, the rich findings provided by qualitative research are a goldmine for improving the quality of our patient care.

REFERENCES

1. Beck CT. The anniversary of birth trauma: failure to rescue. Nurs Res 2006a;55(6): 381–90.

2. Beck CT. Birth trauma: in the eye of the beholder. Nurs Res 2004;53(1):28–35.
3. Beck CT. Posttraumatic stress disorder due to childbirth: the aftermath. Nurs Res 2004;53(4):216–24.
4. Polit DF, Beck CT. Nursing research: generating and assessing evidence for nursing practice. Philadelphia: Lippincott, Williams, & Wilkins; 2008.
5. Merleau-Ponty M. The primacy of perception. Evanston (IL): Northeastern University Press; 1964.
6. Husserl E. Ideas: general introduction to pure phenomenology. New York: Macmillian; 1962.
7. Heidegger M. Being and time. New York: Harper & Row; 1962.
8. Merleau-Ponty M. What is phenomenology? Cross Curr 1956;14:59–70.
9. Beck CT. The lived experience of postpartum depression: a phenomenological study. Nurs Res 1992;41(3):166–70.
10. Kuzel A. Sampling in qualitative inquiry. In: Crabtree B, Miller W, editors. Doing qualitative research. Thousand Oaks (CA): Sage; 1999. p. 33–45.
11. Patton M. Qualitative evaluation and research methods. Newbury Park (CA): Sage Publications; 1990.
12. Colaizzi PF. Psychological research as the phenomenologist views it. In: Valle R, King M, editors. Existential phenomenological alternatives for psychology. New York: Oxford University Press; 1978. p. 48–71.
13. Giorgi A. Phenomenology and psychological research. Pittsburgh (PA): Duquesne University Press; 1985.
14. Van Kaam A. Existential foundations of psychology. Pittsburgh (PA): Duquesne University Press; 1966.
15. Beck CT. Reliability and validity issues in phenomenological research. West J Nurs Res 1994;16(3):254–67.
16. Van Manen M. Researching lived experience. New York: State University of New York Press; 1990.
17. Benner P. The tradition and skill of interpretive phenomenology in studying health, illness, and caring practices. In: Benner P, editor. Interpretive phenomenology. Thousand Oaks (CA): Sage Publications; 1994. p. 99–127.
18. Glaser B, Strauss A. The discovery of grounded theory. Chicago: Aldine; 1967.
19. Beck CT. Teetering on the edge: a substantive theory of postpartum depression. Nurs Res 1993;42(1):42–8.
20. Glaser B. The grounded theory perspective II: description's remodeling of grounded theory methodology. Mill Valley (CA): Sociology Press; 2003.
21. Glaser B. The grounded theory perspective III: theoretical coding. Mill Valley (CA): Sociology Press; 2005.
22. Glaser B. Theoretical sensitivity: advances in the methodology of grounded theory. Mill Valley (CA): Sociology Press; 1978.
23. Spradley J. The ethnographic interview. New York: Holt Rinehart and Winston; 1979.
24. Leininger MM, McFarland MR. Culture care diversity and universality: a worldwide nursing theory. Sudbury (MA): Jones and Bartlett Publishers; 2006.
25. Gillespie BM, Wallis M, Chaboyer W. Operating theater culture: implications for nurse retention. West J Nurs Res 2008;30(2):259–77.
26. Harris NA, Hunziker-Dean J. Florence Henderson. The art of open-drop ether. Nurs Hist Rev 2001;9:159–84.
27. Riessman CK. Narrative analysis. Newbury Park (CA): Sage Publications; 1993.
28. Riessman CK. Narrative methods for the human sciences. Thousand Oaks (CA): Sage Publications; 2008.

29. Gee JP. A linguistic approach to narrative. Journal of Narrative and Life History 1991;1:15–39.
30. Labov W, Waletzky J. Narrative analysis: oral versions of personal experience. In: Helm J, editor. Essays on the verbal and visual arts. Seattle (WA): University of Washington Press; 1967. p. 12–44.
31. Burke K. A grammar of motives. Berkeley (CA): University of California Press; 1969.
32. Beck CT. Pentadic cartography: Mapping birth trauma narratives. Qual Health Res 2006;16(4):453–66.
33. Schreiber R, Crooks D, Stern PN. Qualitative meta-analysis. In: Morse JM, editor. Completing a qualitative project. Thousand Oaks (CA): Sage Publications; 1997. p. 311–26.
34. Sandelowski M, Barroso J. Toward a metasynthesis of qualitative findings on motherhood in HIV-positive women. Res Nurs Health 2003;26(2):153–70.
35. Sandelowski M, Trimble F, Woodard EK, et al. From synthesis to script: transforming qualitative research findings for use in practice. Qual Health Res 2006;16(10):1350–70.
36. Noblit GW, Hare RD. Meta-ethnography: synthesizing qualitative studies. Newbury Park (CA): Sage; 1988.
37. Beck CT. Postpartum depression: a metasynthesis. Qual Health Res 2002;12(4):453–72.
38. Sandelowski M. Rigor or rigor mortis: the problem of rigor in qualitative research revisited. ANS Adv Nurs Sci 1993;16(2):1–8.
39. Lincoln Y, Guba E. Naturalistic inquiry. Newbury Park (CA): Sage Publications; 1985.
40. Guba E, Lincoln Y. Competing paradigms in qualitative research. In: Denzin N, Lincoln Y, editors. Handbook of qualitative research. Thousand Oaks (CA): Sage Publications; 1994. p. 105–17.
41. Whittemore R, Chase SK, Mandle CL. Validity in qualitative research. Qual Health Res 2001;11(4):522–37.

Reading and Evaluating Theory in a Research Publication

Kay C. Avant, RN, PhD, FAAN

KEYWORDS

• Theory • Research • Practice • Theory/research interaction
• Interpreting theory

This article is designed to help clinical nurses understand how theory is built, how it is related to research, and how and when theory is used in research publications. It will also help nurses understand how to interpret whether a theory was used appropriately in a study. It is neither a comprehensive treatment of theory development nor a discussion of the need for the use of theory in nursing science, although both are important. The purpose of this article is to help busy nurses "get on with the job" of interpreting evidence from research and evaluating that evidence for soundness so they can use it in practice.

THE BUILDING BLOCKS OF THEORY

Theories are not mysterious or difficult to understand. They are simply a structure of relationships that help us to understand something. They are built up like any other structure. Theories are built from concepts. Concepts are ideas in our minds that represent categories of our experiences. When we attempt to communicate our ideas we use language, usually nouns or noun phrases, to express those ideas. When we are small children we have a limited vocabulary of terms to express our ideas. As we grow and become more sophisticated, our ideas and our language to express those ideas become more sophisticated as well. Language also develops and matures to include real, tangible, and manifest concepts and increasingly includes abstract, latent, and intangible constructs.

The terms that we use to describe practice are also concepts. When we see that those concepts are related, we form statements, like hypotheses, to express how the concepts are related. When there is more than one relational statement about the same thing, we have the beginnings of a small theory. Weinert and coworkers'[1] description of the evolution of a conceptual model for adaptation to chronic illness is an excellent example of how a theory is built from concepts in practice. Johnson's[2]

Department of Family Nursing Care, University of Texas Health Science Center at San Antonio, 7703 Floyd Curl Drive, Mail Code 7951, San Antonio, TX 78230, USA
E-mail address: avantk@uthscsa.edu

Perioperative Nursing Clinics 4 (2009) 231–236
doi:10.1016/j.cpen.2009.05.002 periopnursing.theclinics.com
1556-7931/09/$ – see front matter

description of how she constructed the Medication Adherence Model is excellent example of how theory is built from other theories and literature.

When a theory is tested and found to be supported over time, the relationships expressed in the theory become universally accepted as factual. For instance, the germ theory has been supported by research for such a long time that it is considered a set of scientific laws. Virtually no one questions the germ theory now, although when it was first proposed, it was ridiculed by the scientists of the time. That is the nature of good theories. They demonstrate a new way of looking at a phenomenon that provides new insights, stimulates new questions, and sometimes generates controversy. That is how science in any discipline grows.

DEFINING CONFUSING TERMS

The literature is replete with definitions about what theory is, and these definitions are often used inappropriately or interchangeably and can be confusing. For the purposes of this article, I will define some theory-related terms and try to clear up some of the confusion.

The first three confusing terms are *theory, theoretical framework,* and *conceptual framework*. Many authors use these terms without specifying how they are using them. I will give specific definitions for each term herein; however, the important thing to remember is that they describe virtually the same thing but at different levels of specificity.

A *theory* is an internally consistent group of relational statements that presents a systematic view about a phenomenon and is useful for description, explanation, prediction, prescription, and sometimes control.[3] This fancy definition simply means that all of the concepts in the theory are related systematically to each other, and the whole set of relationships is about a single phenomenon. A theory basically tells the reader "what's what" or "what works" and "how" depending on whether it is descriptive/explanatory or predictive/prescriptive. The term theory is often reserved for "named" frameworks or ones that have been previously tested.[4]

A *theoretical framework* is also a set of relationships among concepts but is usually less well tested than a theory (or has not yet been tested). The direction of the relationships among the concepts or variables is specified in the theoretical framework just as it is in a theory. Theoretical frameworks often reflect a synthesis of the literature and are generated by the authors for the specific research being reported.[3]

A *conceptual framework* is much like a theoretical framework, but the direction of the relationships is not specified. Conceptual frameworks are used when the author speculates about potential relationships but does not know the actual direction of the relationships they are investigating. In this case, the literature is not sufficient or specific enough to allow hypothesizing about whether the relationships are positive or negative. It is the least precise of the three.[3]

The next term that you may see used interchangeably with the three previous terms is *model*. A model is a graphic, mathematical, or verbal description of a theory that captures the central components of the theory. The terms *theory* and *model* are often used interchangeably, but a model may not incorporate the entire theory, only the most salient parts.[3] For the purposes of the rest of this article, I will use the term *theory* as a shorthand for all of these terms.

Propositions and *hypotheses* are the last two terms that are often confused in discussing theories. Again, these two terms mean similar things but the level of specificity is different. A proposition expresses the relationships among concepts in the theory and may be very abstract. Hypotheses may reflect the same relationships but at a much more specific and concrete level. Hypotheses can actually be tested in a research study because the variables are measurable. The hypotheses in a study that uses a theory or a theoretical/conceptual framework must directly reflect the relationships proposed in the theory.[5] Most quantitative research studies will propose hypotheses to be tested but qualitative studies will not. For a thorough refresher related to qualitative and quantitative studies, the reader is referred to the two articles in this issue by Beck and Holtzclaw, respectively.

THE RELATIONSHIP BETWEEN THEORY AND RESEARCH AND PRACTICE

Fawcett[6] described the relationship between theory and research as a double helix, that is, theory and research are closely tied together. A theory should guide research endeavors and research should test the theory. Both theory and research may arise from practice and should reciprocally inform practice. Research and theory are the means toward the end of solving practice problems. Theory, research, and practice together are the bases for knowledge development. Johnson and Webber[4] believe that theory, knowledge, and research are "applied in clinical situations through reasoning" and through critical thinking that is intentional and goal directed. This reasoning is what enables nurses to recognize patterns of patient data and behavior that are clinically significant and allows them to plan interventions that are safe, effective, and efficient.

Critical reasoning also allows nurses to generate new theory based on the observations and judgments made in the clinical arena. Mark and coworkers[7] suggest that generating theory that leads to high quality, safe patient care is essential if we want to demonstrate nursing's ability to explain not only how and why nursing care is effective but also under what conditions.

These explanations require dissemination or sharing so that more than one nurse or group of nurses can benefit from the knowledge being generated. The article by Girard in this issue expands upon this point. The best way to share knowledge is to publish it in some form. The usual choice is an article in a research or clinical journal, but how is the reader to know how sound the new knowledge being reported is? In the following sections, some suggestions are provided for determining whether the theory portion is sound and trustworthy. Elsewhere throughout this issue are good discussions for determining whether the research is sound and trustworthy.

Discussions about theory are different in quantitative and qualitative studies; therefore, the discussions about theory, if they occur at all in a research report, are usually found in different sections of the article and serve different purposes. The next sections look at what those differences are.

HOW THEORY IS USED IN QUANTITATIVE STUDIES

In quantitative research reports, the theory is usually found in one of two places. It may be presented first as a heuristic or overview to guide the literature review, or it may be presented at the end of the literature review as a synthesis of the literature and a lead-in to the research questions. The theory should reappear in the discussion section at the end of the research report as the author ties the study findings back to the theory to demonstrate whether the research supported the theory or refuted it.

When a theory is used in a quantitative study, it should serve as a general "road map" for the entire study. It will provide the relationships to be tested and, as a result, will have a significant role in the researcher's choices of design for the study, the study sample size, the variables included or excluded, the intervention methods used (if an experimental study), and the analysis technique chosen. Gaffney and Henry's[8] study of risk factors for postpartum tobacco use is a good example of a study using two combined theoretical perspectives to guide the study and the analysis.

When you read quantitative research studies, you need to evaluate how effectively the researcher used the theory in designing the study, selecting variables, developing interventions (if an experimental study), and analyzing the data. In the findings section you should also see that the researcher goes back to the theory to illustrate how the predictions from the theory were supported (or not) in the analysis. You should ask the following questions about the use of theory as you read a quantitative study:[3]

What are the major concepts in the theory?

Are all of the concepts defined adequately enough so you understand what they mean? Does the researcher indicate how the concepts will be measured?

Are the relationships of the theory clearly demonstrated either verbally or graphically?

Are the hypotheses or research questions in the study clearly and directly related to the relationships in the theory?

Do the theory and its components inform selection of the variables and intervention techniques targeted for study?

Are the concepts in the hypotheses measured with instruments that clearly match the definitions of the concepts given?

Is the sample size adequate for the number of concepts measured? The novices "rule of thumb" is at least 10 participants for each concept measured. There are also sophisticated computer programs that can calculate the correct sample size. If the researcher used one of these, it should be clearly identified.

Does the analysis answer the research questions appropriately? (A discussion of appropriate research analysis strategies for research designs is covered by Holtzclaw and colleagues elsewhere in this issue and in any good research textbook.)

Does the researcher refer to how adequately the theory informed the study in the discussion section?

Does the researcher discuss the findings in relation to the theory?

Does the researcher discuss how the theory could be modified, or not, based on the results of the study?

If the author does a good job of providing answers to these questions within the research report, the reader can be fairly confident that the theory was used appropriately and that the findings are trustworthy; however, research findings from a single study are not as trustworthy as the same findings occurring repeatedly in different studies. When you are determining if a theory will be useful in your practice, you should take into account the number of studies that have used the theory and how well those studies supported the theory. The level of confidence in repeated findings of the same relationships is significantly greater than that from one study alone.

HOW THEORY IS USED IN QUALITATIVE STUDIES

In qualitative studies, a theory may or may not used. In fact, in some qualitative methods such as phenomenology, theory is rarely if ever used. The reason for this is that the methodology requirements of such studies are that the researcher put aside previous knowledge and thinking regarding the phenomenon in an attempt to understand it from the participants' perspectives.[9] Theory may be used later in the report to help explain findings from the study or to tie the findings into previous theoretical work. To evaluate the effective use of theory, if it is used in these studies, look carefully at how well the researcher relates the findings from the research to the theory in the discussion section of the study.

In other qualitative methods, such as field research or ethnography, a theory may serve to give an overview of the phenomenon or may guide the interview process or the data analysis. In such cases, the same questions may be asked of the research study as if the study were quantitative. Gance-Cleveland's[10] article on using a school-based support group for adolescents who have had addicted parents is a good example of this type of study.

A theory may be the result of the data analysis, such as in grounded theory research. The main purpose of grounded theory research is to generate a theory describing an underlying social process.[11] It is a particularly useful strategy to use in nursing when attempting to describe some of the processes of client's experiences or of nursing practice. A good example of a grounded theory study is the report of Martsolf and Draucker[12] on how childhood adversity impacts the life courses of clients who have suffered childhood sexual abuse.

When evaluating a grounded theory study, you will want to ask the following questions:

Is the research design sound?

Are the coding and analysis appropriate given the data presented? Does the researcher give you enough evidence of how the raw data were coded and classified into categories that you can feel comfortable that the coding is reliable? Does the researcher provide a detailed discussion of how the coding was validated?

Does the researcher provide a clear and detailed discussion of how the theory arose from the data?

Does the researcher provide a clear and detailed description of the theory itself?

Does the researcher tie the new theory into the research literature reported at the beginning of the study?

If the researcher has done a good job answering these questions, the new theory most likely has been developed appropriately; however, a new theory by its very nature has no empirical support. It needs to be tested and used in research to determine whether the relationships are valid and reliable. Because qualitative studies usually have small sample sizes, the findings are considerably less generalizable than those from quantitative studies with adequate sample sizes for hypothesis testing. Caution should be used before putting these fledgling theories into practice before they are tested.

SUMMARY

This brief introduction to the use of theory in research was not designed to be a comprehensive review of theory development or analysis. It was designed to provide a simple overview of how theory may be used in research reports and how to determine whether it has been used appropriately. A sound theory should provide new insights about how to solve practice problems. Using theory in practice allows for better understanding of the phenomena of practice, better communication about the phenomena among professionals, and more efficient and effective care.

When theory is used in a quantitative research report, it should provide the reader with a guide or map to show how the study is put together and some predictions to be tested in the study. In qualitative research studies, a theory will more likely be the end result of the study rather than being used as a guide, although it may be used to help develop interview questions or may be discussed post hoc in the results section to explain the findings of the study.

A theory is most reliable and useful when it has been tested and supported over time. When making decisions about applying any theory to practice, it is critical to evaluate not only the theory itself but also the type and quantity of support it has from the research literature. The more sophisticated one is in reading and evaluating theory in a research report, the easier it will be to determine when the theory is ready for use in practice.

REFERENCES

1. Weinert C, Cudney S, Spring A. Evolution of a conceptual model of adaptation to chronic illness. J Nurs Scholarsh 2008;40(4):364–72.
2. Johnson MJ. The medication adherence model: a guide for assessing medication taking. Res Theory Nurs Pract 2002;16(3):179–92.
3. Walker LO, Avant KC. Strategies for theory construction in nursing. 4th edition. Upper Saddle River (NJ): Pearson, Prentice-Hall; 2005.
4. Johnson BM, Webber PB. Theory and reasoning in nursing. 2nd edition. Philadelphia: Lippincott Williams & Wilkins; 2005.
5. Dulock H, Holzemer W. Theoretical substruction: improving the linkage from theory to method. Nurs Sci Q 1991;4(2):83–7.
6. Fawcett J. The relationship between theory and research: a double helix. ANS Adv Nurs Sci 1978;1(1):49–62.
7. Mark BA, Hughes LC, Jones CB. The role of theory in improving patient safety and quality health care. Nurs Outlook 2004;52:11–6.
8. Gaffney F, Henry LL. Identifying risk factors for postpartum tobacco use. J Nurs Scholarsh 2007;39(2):126–32.
9. Oiler CJ. Phenomenology: the method. In: Munhall PL, Oiler CJ, editors. Nursing research: a qualitative perspective. Norwalk (CT): Appleton-Century-Croft; 1986. p. 69–84.
10. Gance-Cleveland B. Qualitative evaluation of a school-based support group for adolescents with an addicted parent. Nurs Res 2004;53(6):379–86.
11. Glaser BG, editor. Examples of grounded theory: a reader. Mill Valley (CA): Sociology Press; 1993.
12. Martsolf DS, Drauker CB. The legacy of childhood sexual abuse and family adversity. J Nurs Scholarsh 2008;40(4):333–40.

Quality Measurement as the Cornerstone of Respectable Research

Robin D. Froman, RN, PhD, FAAN

KEYWORDS

• Measurement • Psychometrics • Reliability
• Validity • The validation process

THE IMPORTANCE OF MEASUREMENT

Research studies, regardless of whether they are qualitative, quantitative, or mixed methodology, are based upon data. These data represent things that have been measured, either objectively (eg, quantifying blood pressure estimates for individuals) or subjectively (eg, collecting an individual's recall of their reaction to being diagnosed with a critical illness). These foundational data create the basis for statistical analysis, hypothesis testing, interpretation of themes, or development of theories about phenomena. As such, the measured data are the underpinning for research studies and are potentially the Achille's heel of the studies.

The term "GIGO" commonly refers to "garbage in, garbage out." GIGO invokes a particularly salient point regarding measurement. Excellent measurement reduces "garbage" and increases the ability to discover truth in research. Poor measurement allows trash to creep into the foundation of research and can reverberate through studies, obscuring the discovery of truth.

For example, a study of the pressure-reducing effects of various mattress overlays[1] could not start until a measuring device to quantify pressures was devised. The researchers discovered that the standard device that had been used to measure pressures associated with different overlays showed no variation when used across various overlays, with individuals of differing weights, or when the device was stomped upon directly. The tool commonly used to measure pressures did not work and was producing garbage data. The researchers developed their own pressure-measuring tool by using an intravenous bag as a diaphragm attached to a closed system using a transducer to measure pressure. They showed that this new tool actually registered different pressures when different weights were applied to it. Confident that they now had a new tool that actually responded to changes in pressure, they were able to address the real research question of interest: which overlay was best

Center for Nursing Scholarship, School of Nursing, University of Connecticut, CT 06268-0026, USA
E-mail address: RDF@vbbn.com

Perioperative Nursing Clinics 4 (2009) 237–244
doi:10.1016/j.cpen.2009.05.010 periopnursing.theclinics.com
1556-7931/09/$ – see front matter

for pressure reduction. If the researchers had not been sensitive to the lack of accurate measurement information from the standard pressure-measuring tool, then they never would have been able to discover real answers to their question of interest.

MAJOR PSYCHOMETRIC INDICATORS FOR QUALITY OF MEASUREMENT

There is a handy formula that helps express where garbage can come from in measurement. The formula,

Observed score = True score + Error score,

or O = T + E, sums it up. In any score measurement, be it blood pressure or weight estimation or a person's score on a driver's license test, part of the score is truth (T) and part is error (E). The goal of good measurement is to increase truth in observed scores to the maximum and to reduce error to a minimum.

Errors in measurement can creep in from a variety of places. For example, errors can come from the measuring instrument itself, the environment, or the person being measured. A leaky bladder on a blood pressure (BP) cuff creates a faulty instrument and leads to error. Noise in the environment can lead to errors in hearing systolic and diastolic sounds in BP measurement. An individual's reaction to a white lab coat during an office BP assessment can falsely raise BP and create an erroneous reading.

There are established ways to estimate error from various known sources. Two general classes of quality indicators for instruments, reliability and validity information, are used during instrument development and validation to estimate the amount of error, and, in turn, truth in measurements. These are called "psychometric estimates" and are used to gauge the quality of instruments. Reliability can most simply be thought of as the consistency of measurement produced by an instrument. The consistency can be over time, raters, alternate forms of the instrument, or other aspects of measurement. Validity can be viewed as the accuracy of the measurements produced. Reliability precedes and is necessary for validity, but it does not guarantee validity. For example, the author had a scale for weighing herself on each morning. It routinely showed 5 to 12 pounds of variation in body weight from one day to the next. That scale was not reliable (consistent) from one weigh-in to the next, and the author replaced it. The new scale consistently gave her a reading of 110 pounds every morning. It was consistent over time, or reliable, in measurement jargon. However, because the author is 5 feet 6 inches tall and wears a size 14 dress, the 110-pound readings might have been consistent and reliable, but they were not accurate or valid. Consistency in measurement is necessary, but it is not sufficient to produce accuracy. A scale that showed the author's weight as well over 150, and only showed a decline in weight after she began dieting and exercise, was the one that was ultimately reliable and valid.

Both reliability and validity evidence are needed to assess the psychometric quality of a measuring instrument. There are multiple types of reliability and validity estimates possible to calculate, each reflecting a different aspect of a measure's quality. The types of reliability and validity estimates commonly used are described next.

TYPES OF RELIABILITY ESTIMATION

Instruments can show reliability or consistency of measurement across numerous dimensions. In describing reliability, the numerical estimate expresses how much of the measurement is consistent and associated with truth in measurement. The remainder, or the reliability estimate subtracted from 1.00, then multiplied by 100 to create a percent, is the amount of error in reliability of the measure.

One reliability estimate of interest is temporal consistency or reliability over time. That form of reliability is known as either "stability reliability" or "test-retest reliability". In stability reliability, error can creep in from changes in measurements over time. Its estimation requires two measurements on the same individual with a lapse of time in between. Scores from the first testing or measurement are correlated with the scores from subsequent measurement (see the article by Owen on statistics for a description of the correlation procedure). The degree to which the measurements agree, expressed as a coefficient ranging from 0.00 to 1.00, is the stability reliability estimate. Complete agreement between the two measurement occurrences would be 1.00. In reality, most stability coefficients range from something greater than 0.00 into the 0.90s. The coefficient can be interpreted most easily as the percent of score that is stabile over time from one measurement occurrence to the other. Thus, higher values represent stable measurement over time.

How high a stability coefficient estimate is good or acceptable for stability reliability? That depends on two things: the interval between measurements and the nature of the thing being measured. Longer intervals show greater change in scores and lower stability in general. When one measures state like characteristics, or things that are naturally liable and variable, the stability reliability is lower than for measures of stable or trait like characteristics. When Chien and Chan[2] were testing the stability reliability of a Chinese version of the "Level of Expressed Emotion" scale to measure expression of emotion by families of people with schizophrenia, the newly translated instrument was administered twice, 2 weeks apart, to the same individuals. Expressed emotion was conceptualized by the scale's authors as being a stable and unchanging characteristic. The two sets of scores from the repeated administration of the instrument were correlated to estimate how reliable, or consistent, the scores were over 14 days. The coefficient estimate of .88 suggests that 88% of the score variation was stable and unchanged on retesting the same group of people, leaving 12% as changes scores, or error in the measurement.

Another dimension of interest for reliability estimation is error across various versions or types of the measuring instrument. This is called "alternate forms" or "equivalence reliability". Here, error can come from the version of a scale or instrument used. To calculate alternate forms equivalence reliability, two forms of a measure must be administered to the same people, and then the matched scores for each person are correlated. When translating an English-language version of a patient satisfaction scale into Spanish, Lange and Yellen[3] needed to document the equivalence of the different language forms of the same instrument. To create that documentation, they found a group of bilingual of individuals who spoke both Spanish and English and had the group complete both language versions of the scale. The scores from the two different language versions, one Spanish score and one English score for each person, were then correlated. The resulting correlation coefficient of .89 shows that 89% of the variation of scores is consistent or reliable across the two versions and supports the equivalence of the alternate language forms of the scale.

Not all such equivalence reliability studies are so supportive of alternate versions of an instrument. Concern for equivalence reliability is important when one measures things such as blood pressure. In such measurement, all BP cuffs are treated as equivalent, as well as considering scores derived from different cuffs as equivalent. Typically, one measures blood pressure on the arm easiest to access, treating an individual's two arms as interchangeable for measurement purposes. Green and Froman[4] checked that assumption of arm equivalence by correlating systolic and diastolic readings taken across left and right arms of the same individual. For systolic readings measured with a sphygmomanometer (manual, auscultatory cuff) the correlation coefficient across the arms was .78; for diastolic readings, the coefficient estimate was .61. Given that the pressure measurements were taken only minutes apart, they should have been roughly the same, but there was 28% error variation in the systolic readings, and fully 39% error in the diastolic readings. That amount of variation between the readings of a physiologic variable that should be consistent across arms suggests less equivalence reliability and more error coming from arm differences than might be tolerable for clinical decision-making.

A third dimension for reliability estimation is across multiple raters or observers and is called "inter-rater reliability". In the case of inter-rater reliability, error can creep in from differences between ratings given by different observers and not from real differences in the thing being measured. To calculate inter-rater reliability, two raters must evaluate and score the same thing, and then the sets of scores are correlated or compared in some way for agreement. Siddell and Froman[5] wanted to know what criteria were used in neonatal intensive care units (NICU) to determine readiness for oral feedings. They collected nurses' reports of the criteria by sending a survey questionnaire to all of the Level II and III NICUs in the national directory. To estimate the observer reliability of the returned data, they asked for the head nurse and at least one staff nurse in each NICU to complete the surveys. The two surveys from each responding NICU were returned in separate envelopes that had been coded for matching by hospital number. The ratings on each or the 25 survey items were compared across the two raters from each hospital to assess the agreement, or inter-rater reliability, across the head nurse and staff nurse respondents. Agreement on the 25 survey questions ranged from 57.6% to 98.4%. The authors set the acceptable level of inter-rater reliability at 75% agreement and visually inspected those five items showing more than 25% error (falling below the 75% agreement criterion).

The last common type of reliability estimation is "internal consistency". This type of reliability is of primary interest in self-reported measures of attitudes or traits that assume responses on all items on the instrument should be relatively homogenous. In practical application, people high on the characteristic of interest should show a pattern of scoring high on all items and those low on the characteristic should have a scoring pattern lower on the items as a group. There are multiple ways to express internal consistency, and this type of reliability goes by many names including Cronbach alpha estimate, inter-item correlation, split-half estimate, or Kuder Richardson estimate. The interpretation of all of these is the same: the numeric statistic estimates the amount of correspondence, or internal consistency, between responses to the items on the instrument. Watson and colleagues[6] recently developed a scale to measure nurses' attitudes toward obesity and obese patients. They intended the self-report items on the scale to all reflect a relatively homogeneous attitude and expected high scores to show more negative attitudes toward obesity and obese patients. They reported a Cronbach alpha internal consistency estimate for the 36 items on the scale as .81, indicating over 80% of the items had common variation or consistency.

TYPES OF VALIDITY ESTIMATION

As noted previously, reliability is a necessary preceding requirement for accuracy, but it does not ensure validity. Validity estimation is conducted separately from reliability estimation, and is often more difficult to document. The difficulty occurs because in many cases there is no "gold standard" for comparison to evaluate accuracy. one can compare a blood pressure cuff reading to a Swan Ganz reading of systolic and diastolic pressures, and, in that case, one can get a pretty good estimate of how accurate the cuff readings are to a measure taken in the chambers of the heart. What is the gold standard comparison for a measure of self-reported quality of life, attitudes toward AIDS patients, or perceived health? In many cases, when one measures attitudes or other latent, not directly observable characteristics, one has to infer the level of accuracy. This is called the construct validity challenge. Remember that a construct is something that one has attached a name to, like quality of life, but that is intangible and doesn't really exist as a directly measurable entity in reality. All of the various types of validity estimates below fall under the general heading of construct validity. The estimates support or detract from evidence of accuracy of measurement of the construct. Within construct validity, there are estimates of content, criterion-related, convergent and discriminate validity, as well as factorial validity.

When there is a range of content to be covered by an instrument, particularly something like a self-report measure of attitude, representative coverage of the entire domain of content is important. Content validity addresses whether items on a measure cover the whole domain, might unfairly emphasize one or more area, or might leave out important content areas of interest. Initial assessment of content validity is often subjective and relies upon reviewing the literature in the area to define the entire domain of content that is relevant and of interest. Content validity is most frequently addressed in a systematic, more objective fashion by securing ratings from expert judges on content adequacy and relevance of items proposed for a measure. A complete description of the procedure for getting systematic, informative ratings from judges is provided in articles by Lynn[7] and Grant and Davis.[8] The experts' ratings are summarized with a content validity index (CVI) that indicates content relevance of the items. The index includes ratings given by all the judges who are deemed expert, and ranges from 0.00 to 1.00. CVI ratings can be improved by eliminating items deemed not relevant by judges, or writing more items based upon judges' suggestions to cover areas of the content that might have been missed originally. In a recent study of development of a measure of diabetes self-management, the authors initially wrote 63 items based upon their review of the literature in the area.[9] They then sought ratings of the relevance and content coverage from seven designated expert judges. Judges' ratings were summarized as a .90 CVI across the 63 items, a good index of content validity. Based upon judges' suggestions, an additional 11 items were written to improve coverage of all the content relevant to self-management of diabetes. Although only 35 of the original pool of 74 items were retained in the final scale, the authors had evidence from the CVI ratings that content validity was supported.

A second approach to construct validity documentation is to show the correspondence of scores on an instrument to some other criterion of interest and relevance. This approach is identified as criterion-related validity, and the criterion can be either simultaneous with measurement or in the future: concurrent and predictive validity respectively. In the case of concurrent validity estimation, another measure that should theoretically show a strong relationship with the measure being developed is administered and scores from both the new and existing measure are calculated. Why would one seek a new instrument if an instrument is already available to measure the same thing? If a newly developed measure is quicker, less expensive, less intrusive, or easier to use, it can adequately replace the existing measure. For example, consider the comparison of the breathalyzer test, which is used by the highway patrol, to blood alcohol levels (BAL) derived from blood draws and lab analysis. The breathalyzer provides an acceptable measure of BAL because it has shown a very high correlation with actual blood analysis during concurrent validity studies. Because the breathalyzer is less intrusive (ie, the person being tested for blood alcohol breathes into a tube and the exhaled breath is analyzed for alcohol content) than a blood draw, is less expensive, and can be administered on the road by a trained individual, the breathalyzer is more commonly used.

An example of a concurrent validity concern can be seen in the analysis by Green and Froman[4] of readings that were taken at the same time from sphygmomanometer blood pressure cuffs and Dinamap oscillatory machines. The sphygmomanometer cuffs are common in outpatient settings because they are inexpensive equipment and easy to maintain. The oscillatory instruments are more commonly used in hospital settings, but the two are treated as equivalent for valid measurement. Unfortunately, the concurrent correlations of readings, across arms for both systolic and diastolic measurement, were reported by the researchers to range from .58 to .78, showing from 28% to 42% error in the accuracy of two supposedly equal, simultaneous readings. Concurrent validity of the two measuring devices was not sufficiently supported in that study.

Criterion related predictive validity approaches are illustrated by the development of Dexa measures of bone density and blood cholesterol screening. In both cases, the interest is not in the present value of scores or readings but in the predictive validity of foretelling development of future osteoporosis or heart disease respectively. In these cases, the validity of the construct measurement is supported by significant prediction of later disease occurrence.

An extension of criterion related validity is seen in the use of convergent and discriminate validity estimates in documenting construct validity. In this case, the instrument developer selects two concurrent criteria: one that should be related to (convergent) the new measure and an additional measure that should be independent (discriminate) from the measure. For example, a new, self-report written scale to assess pre-operative anxiety should probably correlate well with heart rate, blood pressure and even galvanic skin response because those three variables, when elevated, are physiologic indicators of anxiety. By contrast, the self-report written measure should be unrelated to things such as weight, intelligence, age or reading skill. If the anxiety measure correlates highly with any of the latter variables, it might not be discriminating between them and anxiety. In particular, written self-report instruments might have cracks in their validity if they correlate too highly with reading skill or intelligence, thus creating the suspicion of error coming from inability to read or from a smart person trying to "game" the measure.

The final type of construct validity evidence described here is factorial validity. It is widely used and has been claimed by some to be too heavily relied upon to document validity,[10] while others cite it as the most important statistical method for validating the structure of instruments.[11] Factorial validity relies on the statistical methods of factor analysis to show if responses to items on an instrument group together into a single dimension of measurement, or if they show multiple dimensions underlying responses. You might ask how a statistical analysis on its own can document construct validity. It cannot. The use of factor analysis to show validity requires the developer of an instrument to assert an expectation for the construct being measured to be either unidimensional (ie, a single group response pattern) or multidimensional in nature. The statistical method of factor analysis merely allows testing of that expectation by looking at how responses to all items on a scale correlate with each other.

Without delving into the statistical underpinnings of factor analysis, two examples might suffice to illustrate how factorial validity works. Froman and Owen[12] reported on the translation and validation of a self-report measure of choice for interventions in life-threatening situations, the Life Support Preferences Questionnaire (LSPQ). The construct of interest, preference for life support interventions, was hypothesized as being unidimensional and not expected to show differences in choice related to age or disease of the choice situation. The six-item scale includes vignettes in which life support choices are made in cases that differ based on age (pediatric and adult) and disease (chronic and acute) characteristics. On factor analysis of responses, all the items correlated well with each other, showing a single factor, or dimension, with no separation of life support preference specific to age or disease. The factor analysis of the LSPQ showed unidimensionality, supporting the construct definition theorized by the developers.

By contrast to the case of the LSPQ, a different instrument intended to measure health care providers' attitudes toward AIDS patients was hypothesized to have multiple dimensions, some positive and some negative.[13] When responses to the 21 items on that AIDS Attitude Scale (referred to in the examples provided in the article by Owen) were factor analyzed, two clear groupings of items were defined by the correlations among item responses. One grouping, or factor, was composed of items describing positive, empathetic responses to people with AIDS, such as "I would do everything I could to give the best care to patients with AIDS" and "patients with AIDS should be treated with the same respect as any other patient." The second grouping, or factor, was composed of items showing negative attitudes toward AIDS sufferers, such as "I have little sympathy for people who get AIDS from sexual promiscuity" and "most people who have AIDS have only themselves to blame." The two factors were named "empathy" and "avoidance" respectively. They were not just opposite ends of a single continuum; rather, they were two different dimensions. This finding through use of factor analysis showed empiric support for the definition of the construct attitudes toward AIDS patients as having multiple dimensions.

THE ON-GOING VALIDATION PROCESS

Initial reliability and validity documentation allows a new scale or instrument to be published, marketed and used, but the documentation needs to be revisited periodically to make sure its psychometric properties do not drift or decay, much the way a blood pressure cuff needs to be recalibrated periodically to keep it honest. Aside from looking for the reliability and validity evidence described above, users of instruments should also ask if the language or information included on scales might be dated or dulled. A re-evaluation of the Hogan Empathy Scale, a widely used instrument to measure the psychosocial construct of empathy, was conducted 30 years after the initial publication of the measure.[14] The authors of the re-evaluation were unable to reproduce most of the original psychometric reliability and validity estimates previously reported for the scale. For example, original stability results were reported as .84 over 3 months, but re-evaluation showed stability at only .41. Internal consistency was initially reported as .71, but on re-evaluation it was only .57. When responses on the Hogan scale collected from a sample 30 years after its introduction were factor analyzed, the originally reported factor groupings could not be replicated. People had been using the Hogan scale for three decades without critical evaluation of the current credibility of original psychometric estimates. The scale had become dated, possibly because of language and possibly because of changing attitudes. Regardless of the reason, the psychometric estimates from the 1970s were no longer appropriate for the scales use in the twenty-first century.

This last example is given to make one final point: one should not rely on old data to be convinced of the trustworthiness of measures. Some of the reliability and validity estimates described above are easy to calculate given access to statistical analysis. A first step in many research studies is to calculate one or more psychometric estimate for an instrument and compare it to published estimates. That simple step helps detect error and prevent GIGO.

REFERENCES

1. Burns K, Quinn A, Sideranko S, et al. Effects of position and mattress overlay on sacral and heel pressures in a clinical population. Res Nurs Health 1992;15: 245–51.
2. Chien W, Chan S. Testing the psychometric properties of a Chinese version of the level of expressed emotion scale. Res Nurs Health 2009;32:59–70.
3. Lange J, Yellen E. Measuring satisfaction with nursing care among hospitalized patients: refinement of a Spanish version. Res Nurs Health 2009;32:31–7.
4. Green L, Froman R. Blood pressure measurement during pregnancy: auscultatory versus oscillatory methods. J Obstet Gynecol Neonatal Nurs 1996;25:155–9.
5. Siddell E, Froman R. A national survey of neonatal intensive care units: criteria used to determine readiness for oral feedings. J Obstet Gynecol Neonatal Nurs 1994;23:783–9.
6. Watson L, Oberle K, Deutscher D. Development and psychometric testing of the nurses' attitudes toward obesity and obese patients (NATOOPS) scale. Res Nurs Health 2008;31:586–93.
7. Lynn M. Determination and quantification of content validity. Nurs Res 1986;35: 382–5.
8. Grant J, Davis L. Focus on quantitative methods: selection and use of content experts for instrument development. Res Nurs Health 1997;20:269–74.
9. Lin C, Anderson R, Chang C, et al. Development and testing of the diabetes self-management instrument: a confirmatory analysis. Res Nurs Health 2008;31: 370–80.
10. Goodwin L, Goodwin W. Focus on psychometrics: estimating construct validity. Res Nurs Health 1991;14:235–43.
11. Dixon J. Grouping techniques. In: Munro B, Page E, editors. Statistical methods for health care research. 2nd edition. Philadelphia: J.B. Lippincott; 1993. p. 245–74.
12. Froman R, Owen S. Validation of the Spanish Life Support Preference Questionnaire (LSPQ). J Nurs Scholarsh 2003;35:33–6.
13. Froman D, Owen S. Further validation of the AIDS Attitude Scale. Res Nurs Health 1997;20:161–7.
14. Froman R, Peloquin S. Rethinking the use of the Hogan Empathy Scale: a critical psychometric analysis. American Journal of Occupational Therapy 2001;55(5): 566–72.

Making Sense of Published Statistics

Steven V. Owen, PhD[a,b,*]

KEYWORDS

- Statistics • Quantitative methods • Effect size
- Statistical significance • Clinical Significance

I am a statistician. I sweat whenever someone asks me what I do, because my answer often creates a scowl, or rolling of the eyes, or something like "ackk!" If you had a tough time in your introductory statistics course, you probably have "ackk" feelings about numbers, and you might not be looking forward to reading this article any further. Let me promise you this: it will be better than you predict. This article is not about formulas and esoteric rules. I hope to help cut through odd statistical language and strange notations, and to make sense of studies that use quantitative methods.

TYPES OF QUANTITATIVE ANALYSES: DESCRIPTIVE VERSUS INFERENTIAL

A usual way to categorize quantitative statistical methods is descriptive versus inferential. In a study focused on descriptive statistics, the goal is simply to compress and summarize numbers. The researcher is interested in the specific cases, or sample, that delivered the data. For example, the researcher might want to know more about self-help attitudes of breast cancer survivors in Gotham City. She locates 50 participants, her sample, through referrals from a cancer clinic and from local newspaper advertisements. She assesses their attitudes with a widely used questionnaire, and then summarizes the data with some simple statistics. Note that she is not interested in whether her respondents' attitudes are different from those of younger or older women. Neither is she interested in attitudes of women from a different region. She simply wants to describe the data from her sample.

Inferential statistics work from different assumptions. The most important is that data are collected from a sample of participants who come from some larger population. The reason for this distinction is that the researcher wants to be able to make claims about the population without actually collecting data from the whole universe. In short, she wants to infer population characteristics from her sample of data. There are two keys to this inference. One has to do with how carefully a sample is selected

[a] Department of Educational Psychology, University of Connecticut, Storrs, CT 06269, USA
[b] 2420 Toyon Drive, Healdsburg, CA 95448, USA
* University of Connecticut, Storrs, CT 06269.
E-mail address: svo@vbbn.com

Perioperative Nursing Clinics 4 (2009) 245–258
doi:10.1016/j.cpen.2009.05.007
periopnursing.theclinics.com
1556-7931/09/$ – see front matter

and retained, which is part of research design (see the other articles in this issue by Holtzclaw for design, and Menses and Roche for sample recruitment and retention). The second key is the probability value, abbreviated "*P* value," which is a statement about whether the sample data do or do not show an effect. Because *P* values are peppered throughout quantitative studies in every field, it is important to understand a little about what is the *P* value (see later).

Although a published study might concentrate on inferential statistics, it usually contains some descriptive aspects. The first table in an inferential paper is typically a numerical summary that describes the sample (eg, the average age, numbers of each gender, years of education, or other biographic data that were collected). The point of such detailed description is to give the reader a sense about who the sample is and what population it represents. For example, results of a study of persons aged 60 to 85 probably do not generalize to a population that includes 30 year olds. Strictly speaking, the study results should refer to the population aged 60 to 85. How about age 59 or 86? It makes sense to loosen up a little, but beware that loosening up too much reduces a study's credibility. One should pause if the author of the study of the elderly discusses the results as though they referred to adults in general.

TYPICAL DESCRIPTIVE SUMMARIES

Data collected from study participants are sometimes categorical. Categorical data refer to group membership, and the numbers that are attached to groups are meaningless codes; they have no purpose except to identify to which group a person belongs. For example, females = 1 and males = 0; or treatment group = 1 and no-treatment group = 2. One could just as well flip this over, so that females = 0 and males = 1; or treatment group = 2 and no-treatment group = 1. Whatever the group codes, one simple summary is to calculate group percents, such as females (74.1%) and males (25.9%). When the subgroup percentages do not add to 100%, it usually means that some data are missing, as might happen on a mail survey where respondents purposely or accidentally omit items. When authors fail to discuss their own missing data, readers have a harder time figuring out who the sample really is, and what the results really mean.

Table 1 shows a couple of descriptive summaries of some biographic data from a large survey of attitudes toward persons with AIDS (see the article by Froman elsewhere in this issue for a brief description of the survey). The table is typical descriptive output from a popular statistical package. **Table 1** summaries include both the raw counts and the percents for each category. There are large amounts of missing data. A hundred respondents failed to say whether they were male or female, and even more omitted educational information. Imagine how much missing data there might be for sensitive questions! Note that the missing data create different values in the two percent columns. Are females 68.6% or 82.8% of the sample? The "Percent" column shows calculations for all categories including the set of missing values. The "Valid Percents" gives percents only for legitimate categories. Because most researchers do not consider "Missing" to be an actual subgroup in the data, it is usually better to trust the "Valid Percent" numbers.

Percent summaries can also be shown with a graphic device, such as a bar chart (**Fig. 1**) or a fancier "clustered" bar chart with more than one variable (**Fig. 2**). The clustered bar chart, combining gender and highest degree, delivers an important discovery that had been hiding in the frequency summaries of **Table 1**. There are sharp differences in the educational background of males and females, with 95% of the males having graduate degrees. The central variable in this data set is "Attitudes

Table 1
Examples of frequency summaries

Gender

		Frequency	Percent	Valid Percent
Valid	0.00 male	83	14.2	17.2
	1.00 female	400	68.6	82.8
	Total	483	82.8	100
Missing		100	17.2	—
Total		5830	100	—

Highest degree

		Frequency	Percent	Valid Percent
Valid	0.00 doctorate	133	22.8	29.6
	1.00 masters	179	30.7	39.8
	2.00 bachelors	116	19.9	25.8
	3.00 high school	22	3.8	4.9
	Total	450	77.2	100
Missing		133	22.8	—
Total		583	100	—

Toward Persons with AIDS." If the researcher claims that there are gender differences in attitudes, a competing hypothesis is that it is educational background, not gender, which makes the difference. This competing hypothesis would not have emerged by studying variables one at a time (as in **Table 1**).

A pie chart is another graphic device used to summarize categorical data. Although pie charts are straightforward, they are a little clumsier because the viewer must glance back and forth between the colored pie slices and the legend that matches colors to groups. Pie charts also get more confusing as more groups are added. Simple pies, as in **Fig. 3**, are easy to digest. **Fig. 4** shows a more typical pie chart.

Bar and pie charts can give a fast and intuitive summary of group sizes or proportions. Such graphics usually reveal less information than frequency tables do, although the clustered bar graph was an exception. Descriptive summaries, especially graphics, take a lot of precious journal space, so it is common to pile a bunch of descriptive data into a single table.

INTERPRETING MEASURED DATA: HOW DO SCORES CLUSTER?

Whereas the numbers assigned to grouping data are meaningless, other numerical schemes have inherent meaning. In measuring age, attitudes, or Apgar score, higher numbers reflect more of the characteristic. Because measured data often have many possible values, summaries using frequency tables, bar charts, and pie charts create complex messes. Instead, quantitative studies use other numerical summaries commonly familiar. When data are drawn into a frequency distribution, they often pile up in the central region, and thin out on both tails, as shown in **Fig. 5**. No actual data set shows a perfectly normal distribution (the famous bell-shaped outline). In **Fig. 5**, a normal distribution is superimposed, and one can see juts and jags here and there in the data. Overall, however, the age data seem fairly close to an idealized normal distribution. Why should one care? As a distribution grows lopsided, the most common way to summarize measured data, the mean, becomes untrustworthy. With a pretty normal distribution for age, the mean (= 51.06; see **Fig. 5**) is a good summary of how the data cluster toward the center of the distribution.

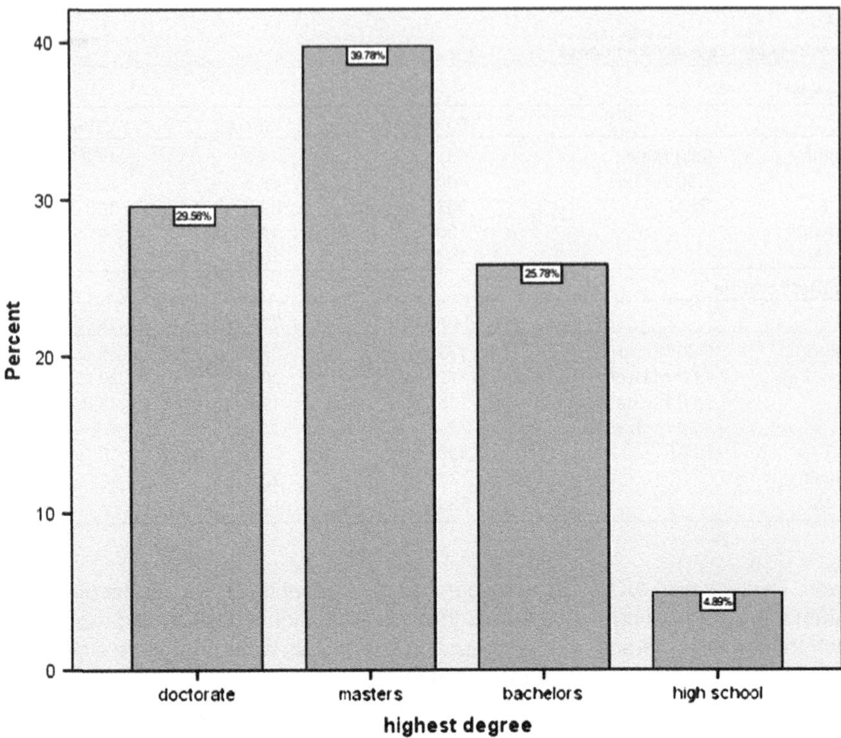

Fig. 1. Example bar graph of educational status.

For an example of how the mean can be distorted, look at responses to one of the items from the AIDS Attitude Scale (described by Froman in another article found elsewhere in this issue). The item is "I have little sympathy for people who get HIV/AIDS from sexual promiscuity." Respondents used a six-point scale to answer this item, with 1 = Strongly Disagree and 6 = Strongly Agree. **Fig. 6** shows that the data for this item had a strong positive skew, with most respondents piling up at Strongly Disagree, and many fewer spreading out on the tail to the right.

Fig. 6 shows that the average score is 2.06, implying that the "typical" respondent circled Disagree"(= 2). Do your eyes tell you a different story about what the "typical" respondent said? I asked the computer to calculate a different version of "typical," the median. Remember that the median score is exactly the halfway point in a distribution, with 50% of the scores on one side of the median, and 50% on the other. The median is 1. The lesson here is that, although the mean is by far the most popular measure of "typical" scores in a distribution, it is vulnerable to skewed data. The median, by comparison, is not affected at all by extreme scores. If someone had mistakenly entered a score of 6000 instead of 6, the median is still 1, but the mean becomes a nonsensical 14.5. Readers should be skeptical of research articles reporting means from highly skewed data.

INTERPRETING MEASURED DATA: HOW DO SCORES SPREAD OUT?

The mean and median are useful summaries of central tendency, simple measures of typical scores. Equally important and reported just as often is an assessment of variability in the distribution of scores. There are several ways to summarize variation

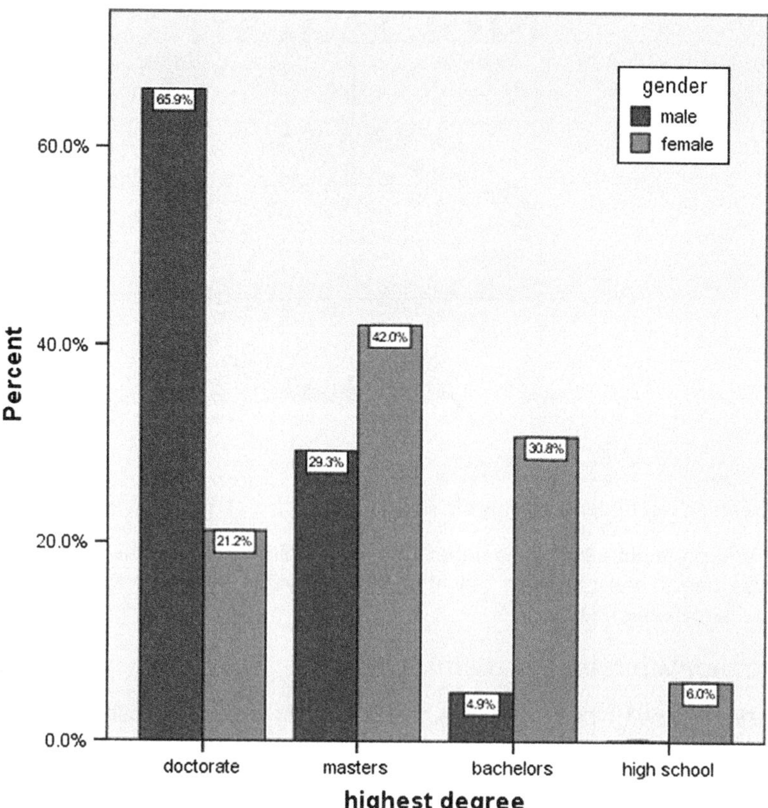

Fig. 2. Example of clustered bar chart.

in scores, but the most widely used is the standard deviation (SD). You might remember using an imposing formula to hand calculate the SD for a small set of data. Possibly you were so focused on following the formula that you forgot (or never knew) the simple meaning of the SD. It is, roughly, the average (standard) distance (deviation) of all scores from the mean. Imagine two distributions with exactly the same mean of 50. If this is the only information you have, you might conclude that the two distributions of data look the same. If I told you that the first one has an SD of 5, and the second has an SD of 10, the pictures are suddenly different. The first distribution has scores fairly packed together, and the second distribution is more spread out. Here is a hint about detecting skewed distributions: when a distribution of scores has an SD that approaches the size of, or is larger than, it's mean, it is guaranteed to be a skewed distribution. See **Fig. 6** for an example of a large SD compared with the mean.

WHAT TO EXPECT FROM INFERENTIAL STUDIES

This section looks at studies that use inferential statistics, whose purpose is to make a statement about a population from a sample of data. All inferential analyses involve a null hypothesis, whether or not the author writes one. The null hypothesis, in its most general form, states that in the population, there is no relationship between specific variables. For example, one might be thinking about a relationship between attitudes toward persons with AIDS and years of clinical experience; or possibly between

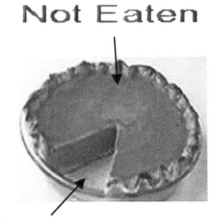

Fig. 3. Everyone can understand this pie chart.

gender and preventive foot care behaviors among diabetics. It is the null hypothesis that gives rise to the common but mysterious *P* value, which is the backbone of statistical significance testing.

INTERPRETING *P* VALUES IN AN INFERENTIAL STUDY

Assume that the null hypothesis is true, that there is no relationship between A and B in the population. When the sample data are analyzed, the *P* value is a statement about

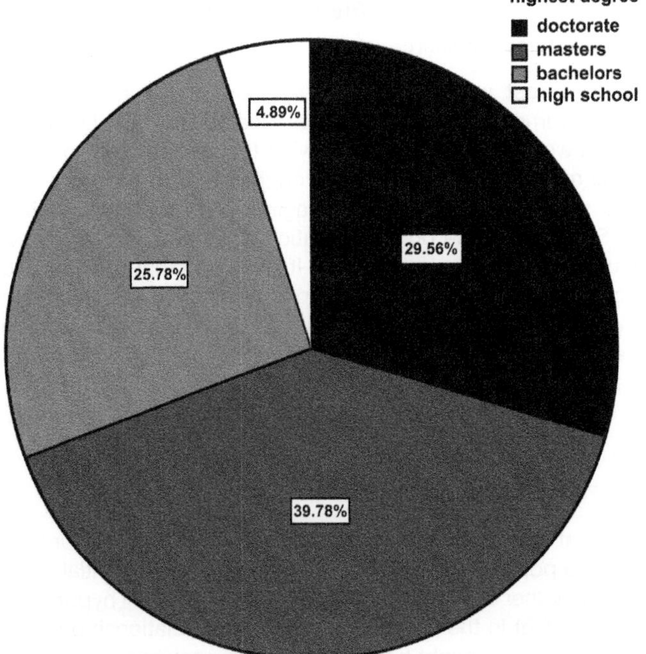

Fig. 4. Example pie chart of educational status.

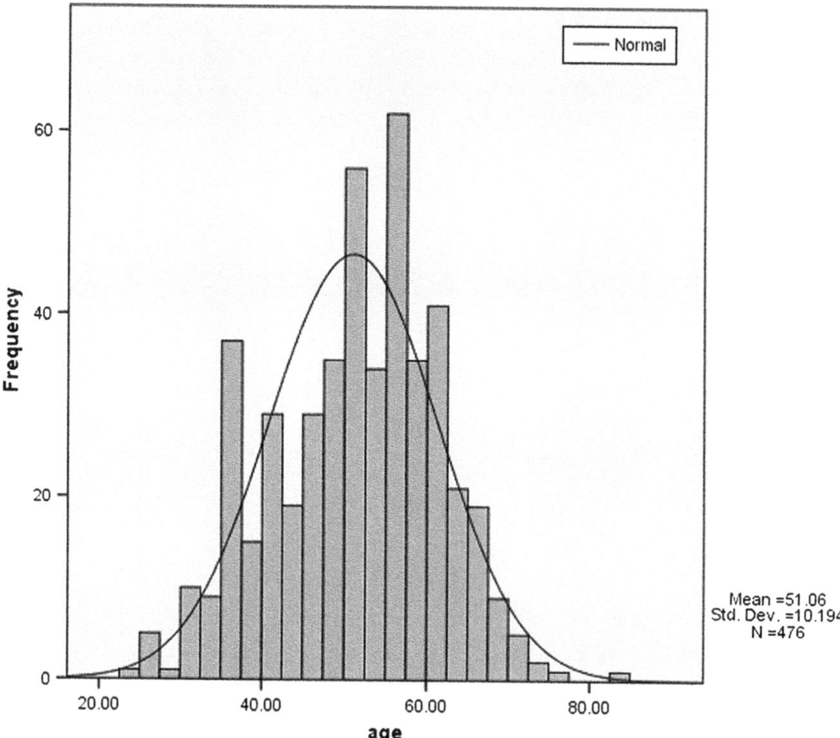

Fig. 5. Frequency distribution for age.

how likely the sample data are, given no relationship in the population. If the null hypothesis is true, what is the probability that the sample data could show whatever pattern is present? If the probability is very small (eg, $P = .02$), it means that the pattern in the sample data is pretty unlikely, given the null hypothesis. The further interpretation is that the null hypothesis should be rejected (ie, there probably is a relationship). Note the word "probably." Although the chances are small, there are sometimes accidental blips in data that cause researchers to claim a particular relationship, when in truth there is no relationship. The opposite problem sometimes occurs: failing to discern an actual relationship. Replication, a fairly unpopular strategy (because researchers and journal editors favor new directions, not the same stuff), is one way to discover whether previous results are blips or genuine.

There have been decades of debate about the use and worth of the *P* value, but it holds a firm place in inferential statistics. It is widely accepted that *P* values equal to, or smaller than, 0.05 signal a significant relationship; statistically significant, but possibly not clinically or practically meaningful. Sample size is responsible for any disparity between statistical and clinical significance.

WHAT AFFECTS THE *P* VALUE?

There are two main influences on the *P* value. One is sample size, which acts like a magnifying glass for perceiving relationships. Large samples create greater "optical" power, so even tiny relationships can be seen. Consider the Nurses Health Study II,[1] which began in 1989 with over 116,000 women enrolled (later subgroups, which gave blood and urine samples a decade later, were also huge, with

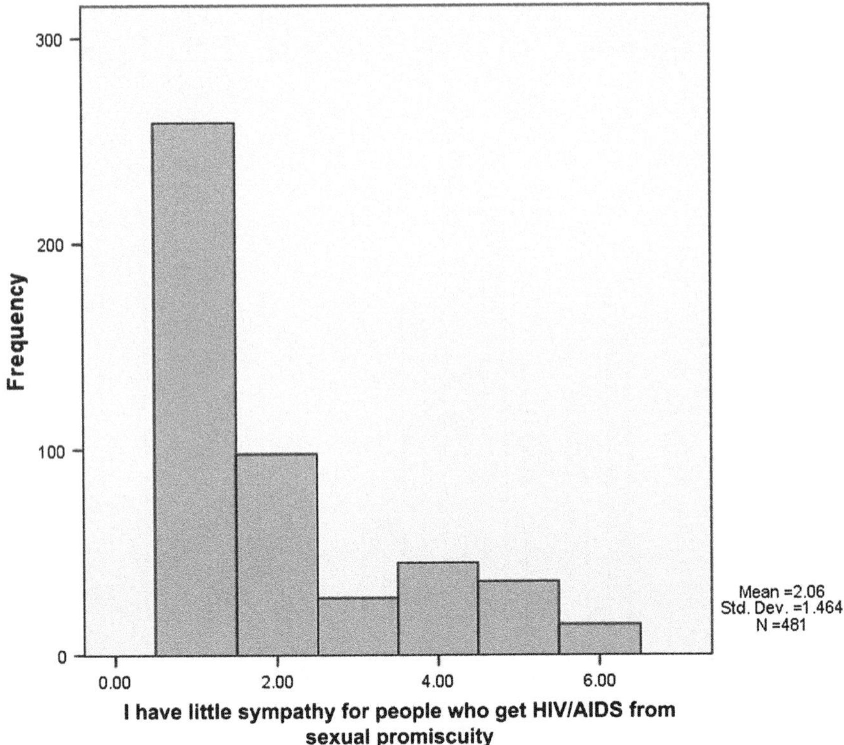

Fig. 6. Frequency distribution for AIDS attitude scale, item 21.

N approximately 30,000). With samples this large, even microscopic relationships can be statistically significant. The problem here is making too much of some of the statistically significant dust motes. By comparison, small samples, often found in exploratory, beginning stages of research, have less power to detect relationships. With a sample size (eg, N = 30) a relationship has to be obvious to the naked eye for a *P* value to be less than or equal to 0.05. Predictably, the small sample problem is that reasonable relationships can evade detection by the significance threshold.

The second influence on *P* is the magnitude of the relationship, usually called the "effect size." Large effects should be easy to detect, no matter what the sample size. Puny effects, however, whether statistically significant or not, should be called puny (researchers prefer more sophisticated terms, such as "trivial" or "not meaningful"). For the last 30 years, there has been increasing attention to reporting effect sizes along with *P* values, and some journals require both for quantitative studies. Because effect sizes are completely divorced from sample sizes, they offer a complementary perspective on study results. At one extreme, it is possible for a study with a large sample to have a raft of statistically significant results, but most of the relationships are ignorable because of their tiny effect sizes. At the other extreme, a small N study might show no *P* value less than or equal to 0.05, but still have important findings because of medium or large effect sizes.

The remainder of this article discusses each main form of statistical analysis and offers guidelines for interpreting effect sizes within the analysis. The effect size guidelines are adapted from Cohen,[2,3] who suggested grouping effect sizes into the crude categories of small, medium, and large. These levels came from Cohen's[2] review of typical effect sizes of published research from social and abnormal psychology. One might wonder whether psychology effect size categories derived more than 45 years ago have anything to do with health sciences research today. Should not modern effect sizes be larger in the health professions, especially medicine, because interventions are stronger and measurements more accurate? That is not the case. Meyer and coworkers'[4] review of over 800 samples shows that effect sizes in the health professions are strikingly similar to those that Cohen found long ago. Indeed, evidence-based practice in health care is sometimes built on very small effects.

Predictably, there are several ways to calculate and report an effect size. The most intuitively simple effect, the squared correlation (r^2) or the squared multiple correlation (R^2), is used here. The squared correlation is intuitive because for any form of analysis, the total variation in scores is always 100%. A statistical analysis shows how much of that 100% variation is explained by some effect. R^2 or r^2 is the proportion of variance accounted for by an effect. With $R^2 = 0.13$, for example, one can conclude that the effect has explained 13% of the variation in the outcome.

COMPARING FREQUENCIES OF TWO OR MORE GROUPS

Frequency counts are used to summarize categories of data. The χ^2 (chi-square) statistic offers a test of whether the various frequencies across groups are different. It can be used with only two groups (eg, frequencies of males versus females in a data set), but that is usually uninformative. It is more interesting to use two grouping variables simultaneously (eg, gender and retirement status [yes/no]). Then, the null hypothesis is that there is no relationship between gender and retirement status. With the AIDS attitude data, comparing the numbers in each of the four groups (males and females, retired or still working), the resulting χ^2 is 0.21, with a P value of 0.65. This is plainly nonsignificant, so the null hypothesis remains in place. Because gender and retirement are unrelated, males and females are equally likely to be retired (or working) in the data set.

If there are only two group frequencies to compare, the χ^2 needs nothing further. If it is significant, one looks at the two frequencies and declares that one group is significantly different from the other. There are usually three or more group frequencies to compare. The χ^2 is an overall test of frequencies: for however many groups, it asks whether there is unexpected variation in the frequencies. In the example using gender and retirement status, there are four subgroups. Because the result was nonsignificant, one is unconcerned about how specific subgroups may differ in size.

Fig. 2 shows what looks like male and female disparities in educational degrees. That comparison is between gender and four levels of education, so $2 \times 4 = 8$ groups. The significance test of these two categories comprising all eight groups gives $\chi^2 = 70.48$, with an associated P value of 0.0000000000000003, so the null hypothesis is tossed out. Reporting a long string of zeros in a P value is not very instructive, and authors usually abbreviate with something like $P < .001$. Sometimes researchers mistakenly write $P = .000$ (instead of $<.001$), because that is what their statistical program reported. But P stands for probability, and probability by definition is never precisely zero.

In any case, the significant χ^2 shows that the two grouping variables, gender and education, are related, but beyond that it is uninformative. It says nothing about which specific subgroups are different from which other groups. The researcher falls back on descriptive detail to explain what the χ^2 means. **Fig. 2** shows that the greatest disparities occur with a much larger proportion of men with doctoral degrees, and a much larger proportion of women with bachelor's degrees.

EFFECT SIZE FOR χ^2

Within the R^2 family, Cramér's φ^2 represents how much variation in one category's frequencies is explained by the other category's frequencies. Cohen's rough effect size suggestions are a little complicated, and depend on the number of groups. For a 2×2 table, the guidelines are small Cramér's $\varphi^2 = .01$; medium Cramér's $\varphi^2 = .09$; and large Cramér's $\varphi^2 = .25$.

It was seen that retirement status could not be predicted by gender in the AIDS attitude data, and the effect size of Cramér's $\varphi^2 = .0004$ confirms the independence of these two categorical variables. For the test of whether gender and educational status were related, Cramér's φ^2 was .16, which, from Cohen's rough guidelines, is a medium-to-large effect.

Reporting effect sizes is far from universal, but it is easy to calculate them with information in a published article. Cramér's φ^2 is a simple derivation, shown in Appendix 1.

COMPARING MEASURED OUTCOMES FOR TWO INDEPENDENT GROUPS

By "independent groups," is meant that respondents show up in one group, but not both. Scanning the AIDS attitude data, one notices that males and females seem to have different backgrounds, with males reporting an average of 14.3 years of professional experience, and females, 16.6 years. There are two versions here of the null hypothesis. One is that there is no reliable difference in years of experience between males and females. The equivalent null is that there is no relationship between gender and years of experience. The test of the null hypothesis is done with a *t* test, the standard two-group approach. This produces a *t* value of 2.07, with $P = .039$. There is a significant difference in experience (and there is a relationship between gender and experience).

What is the magnitude of the effect? Corresponding to the two different forms of null hypothesis, there are two options for effect sizes. One is Cohen's *d* (or a variation, Hedges' g), which refers to the distance between the two means in terms of SDs. This summarizes how different are the groups. The other is the squared correlation coefficient (r^2), which estimates how much of the variation in years experience is explained by gender.

Cohen's rough guidelines are as follows: small = 0.2 SD separating the group means (equivalent to r^2 of 0.01); medium = 0.5 SD ($r^2 = 0.06$); and large = 0.8 SD ($r^2 = 0.14$). In our data, Cohen's $d = 0.25$; the male and female means are a quarter of a standard deviation apart, which is a small effect. Computing an r^2 gives 0.01, still a small effect. If an article gives no effect size, it can be readily calculated, as shown in Appendix 1.

COMPARING MEASURED OUTCOMES FOR THREE OR MORE GROUPS

The *t* test can handle only two groups at a time, so if a researcher has multiple groups, the *t* test becomes clumsy. For example, using the *t* test approach with four groups creates a slew of seven significance tests. The more comprehensive approach here is the analysis of variance (ANOVA). Instead of one *t* test after another, the ANOVA economically assesses all possible combinations at once. The ANOVA test statistic is the *F*-ratio, named after ANOVA's inventor, Sir Ronald Fisher. Like the χ^2, the *F*-ratio is an overall statistic that does not tell exactly which groups are responsible for an overall effect. Unlike the χ^2, there are several follow-up tests that pinpoint where the effect is concentrated. These are called, generally, pairwise comparisons.

The AIDS attitude data contain a subscale called "Avoidance," with an example item, "Patients who are HIV positive should not be put in rooms with other patients." An initial null hypothesis is that there are no differences among Asian, Hispanic, black, or white respondents on responses to the item. With an F-ratio of = 4.70, significant at $P = .003$, one bids goodbye to the null hypothesis. A probe of the overall effect with Tukey pairwise comparisons shows no differences among Hispanic, black, or white respondents. Asians, however, scored significantly higher than other groups on that item.

ANOVA effect sizes may be expressed as either Cohen's f, a measure of how spread out are the group means, or R^2, the squared multiple correlation. Cohen's crude categories are small $f = 0.2$ to 0.5 SD (depending on the number of groups and spacing of means) (minimum $R^2 = 0.01$); medium $f = 0.5$ to 0.9 SD (minimum $R^2 = 0.06$); and large $f = 0.8$ to 1.6 SD (minimum $R^2 = 0.14$).

In the data, Cohen's $f = 0.39$, a small effect. Converting this to R^2, one gets 0.01, small again. The interpretation of the R^2 is that racial-ethnic status accounts for only 1% of the variation in the item scores. Calculating effect sizes from published data is a little more complex, especially with "factorial" ANOVA.[5] Appendix 1 shows how to calculate effect sizes for simple ANOVA designs.

MEASURING CHANGE OVER TIME FOR ONE OR MORE GROUPS

Longitudinal studies are common in the health professions. One often is interested in whether a change between premeasurement and postmeasurement is significant. In the simplest case, a single group is measured on two occasions. The usual statistical assessment of change is the correlated (or dependent) t test, which is variation on the independent groups t test; the formula is adjusted to acknowledge that each participant shows up at each measurement occasion. In complex designs, there may be more than one group measured repeatedly (eg, males versus females measured on two or more occasions). Advanced designs are usually assessed with repeated measures ANOVA.

The formula for calculating a Cohen's d effect size is simple, but it requires knowledge of the correlation between prescores and postscores, which is almost never given in published articles. If a researcher happens to report Cohen's d or Hedges' g, one may use the small, medium, or large effect sizes suggested previously.

Cohen did not write about repeated measures ANOVA designs. Grissom and Kim[5] discuss how to calculate effect sizes from such designs, but the calculations are complex and require more information than is usually given in published articles. If an author gives any version of the R^2 family (omega squared, eta squared, partial eta squared), one can use the "minimum R^2" guidelines mentioned previously.

EVALUATING RELATIONSHIPS AMONG VARIABLES

Relationships between two measured variables are summarized by the simple (or Pearson) correlation, abbreviated as r. Relationships between one measured variable and a collection of others delivers a multiple correlation, or R. This arrangement is typically formed in an analysis called "multiple regression" by having the group of variables predict a single outcome variable. Any sort of correlation is slippery to interpret, for one reason because it refers to a nonlinear scale. For example, the interval between $r = 0.10$ and $r = 0.20$ is not even close to the apparently equal interval from $r = 0.80$ and $r = 0.90$. To simplify the interpretation of r, or R, just square the value, as suggested previously. The squared correlation is now on a linear scale, and the interval between $r^2 = 0.20$ and $r^2 = 0.30$ is identical to the distance between

r^2 =0.45 and r^2 = 0.55. Even better, the squared values represent an intuitively simple idea: the proportion of explained variation.

Fortunately, researchers using correlation (or regression) analysis always report *r* or *R*, and often report the squared values, so the only translation necessary is to use Cohen's rough legends (**Table 2**).

LINKING STATISTICAL RESULTS WITH THE STUDY'S DISCUSSION AND CONCLUSIONS

Large samples are not rare in nursing research, and their advantage is having enough statistical power to detect even tiny effects. A statistically significant tiny effect, however, is not necessarily a meaningful effect. That is why it is important to report and interpret effect sizes alongside *P* values. Because nursing journals do not require discussion of effect sizes, the critical reader may want to calculate unreported effects and consider interpreting them with Cohen's crude guidelines. This seems especially important when an author of a large N study draws deep conclusions based solely on significant *P* values. Examination of the effect sizes may show that some or all of the statistically significant effects have vanishing effect sizes and little clinical use.

A different situation occurs with a small N study showing statistically significant results. Small samples make it hard to detect effects, so if *P* less than or equal to 0.05 is reported, it almost certainly sits atop an impressive effect size. In that situation, it is surprising that a researcher fails to report another signal of success, an impressive effect size.

Calculating effect sizes is more than just fussing with numbers. It is a clinically meaningful balancing weight for the dominance of the *P* value. One day, journals and their readers will regard effect sizes and *P* values as complementary partners.

Finally, the issue of measurement error is possibly as important as *P* values and effect sizes in quantitative articles. Ironically, despite its importance, measurement error is almost universally ignored. In another article in this issue, Froman discusses reliability coefficients, which range in value up to (the impossible) 1.00. Any value lower than 1.00 is a result of measurement error. Most researchers know that high reliability is a good thing, but they fail to connect measurement error with their statistical analysis and conclusions. The principle linking measurement and analysis can be stated simply: measurement error degrades statistical analysis. The corollary is predictable: more measurement error creates more degradation. When only two variables are involved in an analysis, the form of degradation is known: measurement error inflates *P* values, making it harder to declare statistical significance. That, in turn, means that the researcher has a higher risk of ignoring an effect that actually exists. But when an analysis contains more than two variables, the effects are not at all clear, sometimes inflating *P* values, and sometimes deflating them. Still, the message remains. Measurement error creates biased statistical results, which in turn can lead to incorrect conclusions and subpar clinical practice. Journals reporting nursing research often require authors to make some mention of reliability estimates. When one spots

Table 2
Cohen's rough legends

Simple Correlation (r^2)	Multiple Correlation (R^2)
Small = r^2 of 0.01	R^2 of 0.02
Medium = r^2 of 0.09	R^2 of 0.13
Large = r^2 of 0.25	R^2 of 0.26

measurements with weak reliability, one should take the author's conclusions with a large grain of salt, no matter how statistically significant the results or how large the effect sizes.

I have skimmed a lot of quantitative territory in this article, and there is much more to know. I have hinted, for example, that quantitative articles sometimes contain errors or oversights that slip through the peer review and editorial process. For the casual but skeptical research consumer, I hesitate to recommend any text on statistics, all of which are packed with new vocabulary and symbols. Instead, I suggest befriending a statistician, and demanding (gently) that she or he explain some obscure sentence or result in plain talk. A nicely done study can improve clinical practice. As a careful journal consumer, one can also avoid changing clinical practice on the basis of flawed articles.

APPENDIX 1: HOW TO CALCULATE VARIOUS EFFECT SIZES FROM PUBLISHED DATA

For the χ^2 Analysis of Frequency Counts

$$\text{Cramér's} = \frac{\phi^2 = \chi^2}{N(G-1)}$$

where N = sample size and G = smaller of the number of rows or columns.

For the Independent-groups t Test

If there is a clear control or comparison group, then Cohen's formula for *d* is preferred. Without an obvious comparison group (eg, males versus females), Hedges' formula for *g* should be used.

$$\text{The control or comparison group SD} = \frac{\text{the difference between the two means}}{\text{the total sample SD}}$$

$$\text{Hedges'}\ g = \frac{\text{the difference between the two means}}{\text{the total sample SD}}$$

If one would rather calculate r^2, the proportion of total variation explained by the effect,

$$r^2 = \frac{t^2}{t^2 + (N-2)}$$

where t = the published test statistic and N = the total sample size.

For the 1-factor ANOVA

$$\text{Cohen's}\ f = \frac{\text{SD of group means}}{\text{overall SD}}$$

$$R^2 = \frac{F}{F + (N-2)}$$

where F = the published test statistic and N = the overall sample size.

For Correlational Studies

Because the primary statistic from a correlational study is *r* or *R*, all that is needed is to square the value to derive r^2 or R^2.

REFERENCES

1. NHSII. Available at: http://www.channing.harvard.edu/nhs/. 2009. Accessed March 6, 2009.
2. Cohen J. The statistical power of abnormal-social psychological research: a review. J Abnorm Soc Psychol 1962;65:145–53.
3. Cohen J. Statistical power analysis for the behavioral sciences. 2nd edition. Hillsdale (NJ): Lawrence Erlbaum; 1988.
4. Meyer GJ, Finn SE, Eyde LD, et al. Psychological testing and psychological assessment: a review of evidence and issues. Am Psychol 2001;56:128–65.
5. Grissom RJ, Kim JJ. Effect sizes for research. Mahwah (NJ): Lawrence Erlbaum; 2005.

Recruitment and Retention in Clinical Research

Karen Meneses, PhD, RN, FAAN*, Cathy Roche, BSN, RN, FAAN

KEYWORDS

• Nursing • Recruitment • Retention
• Clinical research • Databases

Recruitment and retention of participants in clinical research is a process, not an event. Recruitment and retention can either "make or break" the success of a research study. Recruitment and retention strategies go "hand in glove" with one another and should be considered one of the most vital aspects of the day-to-day conduct of clinical research. Successful recruitment and retention strategies guide the enrollment of the very first research participant and ultimately lead to the final number of total research participants secured. Successful strategies result in adequate statistical power leading to firm study conclusions. Unsuccessful strategies can increase day-to-day costs of clinical research, limit study efficiency, and ultimately threaten the internal and external validity of study results.

Recruitment is defined as the process of identifying and enrolling volunteers for participation in a research study. Retention is the ability to maintain individual participation throughout the duration of the research study. Recruitment and retention are enormously vital aspects of clinical research. This article reviews the process of identifying and enrolling participants for recruitment; describes regulatory requirements influencing subject recruitment; discusses special considerations in the recruitment of children, minorities, and at risk individuals; describes the process of participant retention; describes the utility of tracking databases; and explores clinical nursing roles and responsibilities in recruitment and retention in clinical research.

PROCESS FOR IDENTIFYING AND ENROLLING PARTICIPANTS FOR RECRUITMENT

As stated earlier, recruitment is defined as the process of identifying and enrolling volunteers for participation in a research study. The emphasis in the definition of recruitment is on "process."

School of Nursing, University of Alabama at Birmingham, 1530 Third Avenue South, GM029, Birmingham, AL 35294, USA
* Corresponding author.
E-mail address: menesesk@uab.edu (K. Meneses).

Perioperative Nursing Clinics 4 (2009) 259–268
doi:10.1016/j.cpen.2009.05.001 periopnursing.theclinics.com
1556-7931/09/$ – see front matter

Identifying Volunteers

The process of identifying volunteers for participation in research starts with thinking out loud in constructing the research proposal. Investigators must have basic information about the target population. Details such as the type of participant needed for the study must be specified. These details include, but are not limited to, the age, gender, type of characteristic or condition (eg, preoperative, postoperative, post hospitalization), disease (eg, cancer, heart disease, diabetes, stroke, hypertension, osteoporosis), health problem (eg, pain, sleep disturbance, nutritional deficit), and relationship (eg, patient, caregiver, parent, sibling) of participants. The greater the specificity an investigator has in delineating the characteristics of the target population, the better the process of identifying potential participants for the study.

Once the details of the target population are specified, the next step in identifying the target population is adding details about study eligibility, including inclusion and exclusion criteria and racial and ethnic diversity. For example, let us take the variable of age as an inclusion or exclusion criteria. Age must be specified with explicit rationale for such a decision. If the target population is older women with diabetes and heart disease, the age of the older women must be defined. Is older age defined as 55 years and older with an upper limit or age 55 years and older with no upper limit? Is older age defined based on Medicare criteria of 65 years and older? Defining the variable of age makes a huge difference in identifying participants.

Enrolling Volunteers

The second part of recruitment is the process of enrolling volunteers. This process is highly detailed and includes the following steps: (1) determining how many participants are available for recruitment, (2) determining a viable recruitment plan, (3) using levels of screening for participation, (4) exploring barriers to participant enrollment, (5) examining factors that contribute to likely enrollment, and (6) finding potential participants through various advertising methods. Unfortunately, investigators have traditionally been cavalier in overprojecting the number of participants available for enrollment. An overly zealous and mistaken assumption that the majority of eligible participants will likely enroll is a huge and costly error once enrollment begins.

Determining the number of participants available

Determining the number of participants available for recruitment may be easy or very difficult. If a sampling frame is available, the process is facilitated. A sampling frame is the actual list of potential participants. For example, in the measurement article in this issue, Froman refers to a researcher surveying level II and level III neonatal intensive care units (NICU) as to practice. Enrolling these participants was made easier through use of a sample frame or list of all registered level II and III NICUs in the United States. Referring to that sample frame defined the target population from which to draw. Unfortunately, sample frames are often unavailable. If one were to consider enrolling homeless people or the caregivers of Alzheimer's patients in a study, there is no sample frame or list of such individuals to draw from.

Calculating the accessible sample often begins with reviewing existing data. For example, identifying the magnitude of a particular condition such as breast cancer within the United States can begin with consideration of publicly available Surveillance Epidemiology and End Results (SEER) federal data from the National Cancer Institute.[1] Drilling down to the total number of newly diagnosed individuals with breast cancer within a specified county or within a particular health care setting takes additional fact finding. If an investigator wishes to enroll a population-based cancer sample from a state, either SEER data must be identified or the state in question must collect such data and have the data publicly available. On the other hand, if an investigator wishes to enroll participants from a health care setting, the investigator must establish and maintain contact with the health care setting to gain access to the total number of individuals with newly diagnosed breast cancer.

Determining a viable enrollment plan

Once the target population is identified, the next step in the process of enrolling participants is determining a viable enrollment plan. This plan generally includes the total number of participants required for enrollment, a regular enrollment schedule (eg, weekly, monthly, bimonthly, or quarterly), and a projected estimate of attrition. The enrollment plan should be discussed at regular research team meetings with modifications made as necessary. At the very least, a monthly check of participant enrollment is recommended so that modifications can be made sooner rather than later. The element of time has a way of slipping away quickly, leaving investigators in the unenviable position of reporting results of a statistically underpowered study due to a smaller than hoped for sample. McNees and colleagues[2] discuss a simple technique, CuSUM (CUmulative SUMmation), to help researchers track changes in recruitment over time.

Levels of screening

Incorporating levels of screening before enrollment may be helpful in securing a retainable population of participants. For example, a self-referred potential participant may be asked to first call a phone number and be initially screened during a telephone interview. Second, the potential participant could be asked to attend a group or individual study orientation session where study goals and participant expectations are discussed. Consent forms may be distributed in the orientation meeting. Many institutional review boards (IRBs) request that a potential participant have at least 24 hours to consider a study before agreeing to participate. Third, a potential participant could be asked to schedule an individual consent signing session at which baseline data could be collected after the consent has been signed. Finally, potential participants could be scheduled for the final enrollment or randomization visit during which they would present to enroll or be randomized into the study. The multiple screening levels are designed first to realistically present the study benefits and burdens without minimizing burdens or overemphasizing benefits. Second, the multiple screening levels give the researcher time to develop trust and credibility with the potential participants. Third, multiple screening levels allow the researcher to identify "red flags" or potential barriers to successful participation. For example, if a participant does not present for a scheduled study screening visit, it may indicate a future retention or participation problem if enrolled. Dedicating adequate time and funds to recruiting and screening may alleviate future retention problems.

Factors fostering enrollment

Many factors foster participant enrollment. Perhaps the two most vital factors are the individual's commitment to the study aims and objectives and their passion to help others in a similar situation. These two key factors help participants to weather the time and resources needed to maintain study participation. In today's economy, another unstated factor that stimulates people to participate in research projects is the potential for receiving reimbursement for time spent or care while enrolled. Individuals with altruistic views about the overall good of the research enterprise express strong commitment to enroll in a study, especially if they are familiar with the study targets, such as having a mother with breast cancer or a spouse with Alzheimer's disease. Strong motivators for study enrollment include the costs of laboratory or x-ray studies that may be covered by the research, access to investigational agents such as drugs that may confer benefit, and consistent follow-up regarding one's health problem or health diagnoses when compared with usual care. Whatever the reason motivating participant enrollment, it is helpful to elicit the participant's reason or rationale before study enrollment. The rationale can be used as a motivating force for continued retention in a study, particularly if the study is a longitudinal clinical intervention trial.

Factors hindering enrollment

Barriers to enrollment are many and varied. For example, the individual may not have any interest in the study. A complete noninterest and noncommitment is perhaps the easiest "no" for an investigator to understand. There is no persuasive support for convincing an individual to consider otherwise. A no answer is nonnegotiable. Other barriers that are generally nonnegotiable are the inability to commit based on time, resources, or other competing commitments (eg, family or work responsibilities) and fear of the ramifications of the treatment or complications inadvertently occurring.

Effective recruitment plans include anticipating recruitment barriers and addressing those barriers before recruitment. Possible barriers related to participant referral can include a lack of knowledge about the study, a lack of timeliness in referring potential participants to the study, and clinic staff too busy or unwilling to make referrals. Barriers related to potential participant recruitment can include transportation difficulties, travel distance, lack of child care, the study hours of operation, reluctance to participate in research, the cost of participating (travel, parking, and child care), and the lack of time.

Fixable barriers to enrollment may include transportation costs to and from the research and assistance with child care or other family care responsibilities. These barriers can best be identified at the study outset so that an ongoing strategy to overcome and manage such barriers can be developed.

Study announcements

Methods for reaching potential participants through advertisement and announcements are varied. Announcements for study enrollment include a wide variety of methods and combination of methods such as print materials (eg, posters, mail, newspapers), telephone, media (eg, newspaper and radio advertisement), direct community-based recruitment, and, more recently, electronic and Internet-based methods of recruitment. Each method of study announcement has its own advantages and disadvantages, and there is no specific method preferred over another; however, the most important aspect to consider is the match between where the potential participant is located and the method of study announcement. For example, study announcements using flyers or print materials can be given directly to potential participants who are easily accessible. Radio and television advertisements are more expensive but may engage a hard to reach target population such as Spanish-speaking groups. Im and Chee found their potential participants were geographically dispersed across the globe, necessitating an electronic Internet-based study announcement.[3] Recruitment strategies via the Internet, YouTube, or Podcast messages may appeal to a younger, more technology savvy target audience.

REGULATORY REQUIREMENTS INFLUENCING RECRUITMENT

Three regulatory requirements influence direct access to research participants. These requirements consist of a health care system's IRB and federal HIPAA (Health Insurance Portability and Accountability Act) privacy regulations.[4] The third regulatory requirement influencing recruitment governs gender, minority, and child status and is explicit to research studies supported by the National Institutes of Health (NIH).

The mission of an IRB is to protect the rights and welfare of human subjects involved in research. In the United States, any institution that conducts research using human subjects must adhere to the ethical principles expressed in the Belmont Report, the document that guides IRB practices. The Belmont Report contains three basic principles: (1) respect for persons (refers to the individual's ability to make a voluntary decision to participate), (2) beneficence (refers to the individual's benefit in research participation), and (3) justice (also known as fairness). These ethical principles must be adhered to by the study investigators in a research project. All research involving human subjects must receive approval from an IRB of the institution in which subjects will be recruited for the research.

Federal HIPAA privacy regulations were enacted in 2003. These regulations were not specific to research, per se; however, the interpretation of the privacy rule limited access to participants for enrollment in clinical research. Investigators must preplan recruitment activities that are consistent with HIPAA regulations and include this information in IRB applications. For example, investigators cannot directly access Protected Health Information (PHI) of potential participants nor approach them directly in a clinic or hospital setting that is considered a "covered entity." A covered entity is a health care provider, health care plan, or health care organization that conducts transactions in electronic form. Information about covered entities may be found at: http://www.cms.hhs.gov/HIPAAGenInfo/Downloads/CoveredEntitycharts.pdf.

Investigators must first identify what types of PHI are needed, the possible uses, and disclosures for research purposes in the IRB application. Only after receiving IRB approval can investigators approach participants. Another example is prescreening of potential participants for a study. A HIPAA Waiver of Authorization must first be obtained before participant contact.[4]

All NIH-supported studies are expected to include women, children, and racial/ethnic diversity. NIH-supported studies define children as persons under the age of 21 years. Women, children, and diverse racial/ethnic groups are expected to be included in studies unless there is a strong statement provided regarding the scientifically based rationale for exclusion. For example, children can be logically excluded in a study of breast cancer because the disease is extremely rare in children. Women can be excluded in prostate cancer studies because of the obvious reason that, biologically and anatomically, females are not born with a prostate. If a study specifically targets Hispanics with diabetes based upon their specific language and culturally based barriers to effective management, non-Hispanic participants might rationally be excluded from the enrollment.

SPECIAL CONSIDERATIONS WHEN RECRUITING CHILDREN

Children are a vulnerable population, and the US Department of Health and Human Services Office for Human Research Protections (OHRP) has written guidelines to protect children as research participants. The Protection of Human Subjects (2005) clearly defines children as "persons who have not attained the legal age for consent to treatments or procedures involved in the research" (as quoted in 45 CFR § 46.102). The actual laws vary from state to state in terms of at what age and under what conditions a child has legal authority to consent as an adult. Recruiting children for clinical research requires attaining permission on many levels to ensure that children are protected in light of their vulnerability. Risk versus benefit is considered in all vulnerable populations, such as children, before gaining approval for the study.

When obtaining permission for a child to participate in research, a parent or guardian must first grant permission or consent for the child to take part in the research. Second, the child must agree to take part in the study, defined as assent. The Protection of Human Subjects states (as quoted in 45 CFR § 46.102) "assent means a child's affirmative agreement to participate in research. Mere failure to object should not, absent affirmative agreement, be construed as assent." Assent must be informed, voluntary, and not coerced.

Assent must be not only age appropriate but also developmentally appropriate for the child. Meaux and Bell discuss strategies for ensuring voluntary assent.[5] These strategies include using discussion and a variety of media such as books, models, and videos for communication study purpose, procedures, risks, and benefits. Having a child sign an assent form separate from the parental consent form is recommended by many IRBs. To facilitate voluntary participation and maintain noncoerced assent, special consideration must be given to the incentives provided to children.

Recruiting adolescents for research participation involves not only all of the special considerations necessary for recruiting children but also specific age and developmental related challenges. Typically, adolescents are busy with school, extracurricular activities, and jobs, limiting their time for research participation. Privacy concerns are also important to adolescents. Because research involving adolescents requires parental consent as well as individual consent, the adolescent may fear that sensitive information may be disclosed. Logsdon and Gohmann identified lack of transportation and obstacles involving obtaining parental consent as potential barriers to female adolescent recruitment.[6] Awareness of special recruitment considerations for children and adolescent populations enables the researcher to plan, design, and target recruitment strategies specifically for those populations.

RECRUITING MINORITY AND SPECIAL POPULATIONS

Recruitment of special populations, particularly at risk minority populations, requires sensitivity, additional time, and community support. Barriers to recruitment of minority populations have been historically known in the African American population since exposure of the Tuskegee Syphilis Study and the procedures used unknowingly.[7] The unfortunate and enduring consequences associated with Tuskegee within the African American community are basic mistrust of researchers, feelings of being used and abused by those in power, and racial inequalities in research outcomes.

Specific guidelines must be followed when recruiting prisoners into a study. Local IRBs must have a prisoner representative during the review of any protocol targeting a prisoner population. On the other hand, when an enrolled participant becomes incarcerated, all communication and research activity with that participant must cease immediately and the IRB must be notified. If the research team decides that it is worthwhile to continue contacting the incarcerated participant, two steps must be taken. First, an amendment to the protocol must be submitted to the IRB briefly describing why and how the participant will be contacted. It is understood that permission to contact the prisoner will be granted only after certification from the OHRP is obtained from the IRB. Second, it may be necessary to secure permission from the warden of the prison to have contact with the prisoner. This permission can be accomplished while still maintaining confidentiality because the warden does not need to know which prisoner is being referred to in the request. It is helpful to also contact the mail room at the prison to find out exactly how to address the envelope. If a participant becomes lost to follow-up, it is helpful to check the Federal Prison Web site (http://www.bop.gov/iloc2/LocateInmate.jsp) to see if the participant has become incarcerated.

Other barriers are reported in minority populations,[8] special populations,[9–11] and longitudinal intervention research.[12,13] These barriers continue to present challenges in study recruitment across all types of clinical research. Special considerations must be taken into account in recruitment of at risk populations.[11,14,15] For example, the research team must be culturally sensitive and anticipate the needs of minority individuals when recruiting from these special populations. Specific representation on IRBs is sometimes required for access to these at risk populations (eg, prisoners). Language barriers can be addressed by having translators or individuals fluent in the language of the minority population.

RETENTION STRATEGIES IN CLINICAL RESEARCH

Retention is the ability to maintain individual participation throughout the duration of the research study. Successful retention begins with well-planned targeted recruitment strategies. When trying to determine the best methods of recruitment and retention, researchers must consider the target population and assess the gatekeepers of that population. Gatekeepers are defined as those individuals who control access to the target population. For example, if an investigator is trying to recruit school-aged children, one might consider establishing a partnership with schools to facilitate recruitment of children for research. Community Health Advisors have been used in a variety of studies not only to gain access to a specific population but also to be trusted advocates for research participants. Partnering with various groups within a community, such as churches, schools, and other organizations, may provide access to desired populations. Gaining access means gaining trust and credibility with the gatekeepers.

Effective retention plans begin with effective recruitment strategies. First impressions make a difference in recruitment and retention. The first person the potential research participant comes in contact with must be credible, organized, caring, and knowledgeable about the research.[16] Study personnel must have excellent interpersonal skills with the ability to quickly establish rapport and convey concern and respect for the potential participant.[17]

Retention strategies must be well planned, well funded, and have an adequate number of staff members to devote the time necessary to retention. Many times the study design and the intervention are well planned, but the overall study is not successful due to the unrealistic expectations of retention.

Robinson and colleagues[18] conducted an extensive and systematic review of the literature related to key strategies in retention of study participants. They examined over 3000 citations of which 21 studies were eligible for inclusion. The investigators identified 368 abstracted strategies that they grouped into 12 themes. Key themes included the following:

- Involving the community in the study design, recruitment, and retention
- Creating a study identity for participants
- Placing importance on the characteristics, training, and management of study personnel
- Explaining study requirements and details such as a participant timetable and length of time for study participation
- Having a systematic method for contact and appointments
- Providing reminders of appointments for study participation
- Minimizing participant burden
- Describing study benefits
- Giving financial incentives
- Reimbursing for research-related expenses such as taxi fare and child care during study visits

Giving nonfinancial incentives such as tokens of appreciation (eg, coffee mugs, pens, refrigerator magnets)

Having detailed tracking methods with particular attention to managing participants who may be lost to follow-up

TRACKING DATABASES

Tracking databases are particularly useful when managing the process of recruitment and retention. Tracking with a database on an intranet network allows multiple research users to assess where participants are in the recruitment and retention pipeline. Microsoft Access is a generic database that can be tailored to the particular needs of a research study. During the recruitment process tracking reports can assist the researcher with identifying the status of the recruitment efforts. Tracking reports can summarize successful referral sites and indicate participants recruited and the number not recruited. Tracking reports can provide useful information about why potential participants were not recruited; this information allows study staff to analyze their recruitment strategies and rate the progress toward recruitment goals.

An effective tracking system is crucial for the retention process. Important contact information can be entered into tracking databases and updated by research team members as needed. Entering contact information and a description of the outcome of the contacts into an electronic database is more efficient than sorting through multiple paper forms housed in only one location. Noting the outcome of each contact is important when tailoring retention efforts to the individual needs of participants. Cotter and colleagues[12] indicate that relatives and family friends appear to be the best references for locating participants.

Participants' names, study identification, addresses, phone numbers, appointment dates, missed visit dates, and reasons why a visit was missed can all be recorded in a tracking system. A well-designed tracking system can help prevent participants from "falling through the cracks." Regular research team meetings aided by a tracking system report can facilitate retention. Current strategies can be assessed, and the research team can discuss strategies that are not working and redirect their efforts to more fruitful recruiting efforts. Monitoring recruitment and retention effectiveness is necessary not only to contain cost but also to alert the research team to potential retention risk participants. The earlier a potential retention risk is identified, the sooner the team can use specific individualized retention strategies to prevent attrition. For example, when participants have missed a study visit, the sooner they are called and rescheduled, the more likely they will remain engaged in the study. Diligent and persistent tracking procedures can help to enhance participant retention.

CLINICAL NURSING AND RESEARCH PARTNERSHIPS IN RECRUITMENT AND RETENTION

Clinical nurses who work in partnership with the research team can make tremendous contributions to the recruitment and retention process.[19] For example, clinical nurses have the most day-to-day contact with the target population of clinical research. They know the characteristics of potential participants and can help investigators identify and enroll participants. Hiring clinical nurses as research team members contributes to the successful process and outcomes of recruitment and retention. Clinical nurses can "speak the language" of patients and provide a tremendous advantage in the preparation, submission, and ongoing annual review of IRB and other regulatory requirements. Clinical nurses can also engage communities who represent the population of interest and can maintain contact with key community leaders. Clinical nurses have developed a clinical research management track in schools of nursing, developing key roles in participant retention in longitudinal trials and management of tracking databases to aid in long-term retention.

SUMMARY

Recruitment and retention of participants in clinical research stresses a process orientation rather than a single event. Recruitment and retention strategies make the essential difference between disappointing or limited study results and meaningful, statistically sound, and representative results. Successful recruitment and retention strategies can steer the enrollment of the first research participant and ultimately lead to the total number of participants available for study.

REFERENCES

1. SEER, Surveillance, Epidemiology and End Results. Available at: http://seer.cancer.gov/popdata/download/html/.
2. McNees P, Dow KH, Loerzel VW. Application of the CuSum technique to evaluate changes in recruitment strategies. Nurs Res 2005;54(6):399–405.
3. Im EO, Chee W. Issues in protection of human subjects in internet research. Nurs Res 2002;51(4):266–9.
4. Wipke-Tevis DD, Pickett MA. Impact of the Health Insurance Portability and Accountability Act on participant recruitment and retention. West J Nurs Res 2008;30(1):39–53.
5. Meaux JB, Bell PL. Balancing recruitment and protection: children as research subjects. Issues Compr Pediatr Nurs 2001;24(4):241–51.
6. Logsdon MC, Gohmann S. Challenges and costs related to recruitment of female adolescents for clinical research. J Pediatr Nurs 2008;23(5):331–6.
7. Dawson E. The protection of human subjects: the Tuskegee study. Maxwell Rev 1974;10(2):49–56.
8. Gilliss CL, Lee KA, Gutierry Y, et al. Recruitment and retention of healthy minority women into community-based longitudinal research. J Womens Health Gend Based Med 2001;10(1):77–85.
9. Grap MJ, Munro CL. Subject recruitment in critical care nursing research: a complex task in a complex environment. Heart Lung 2003;32(3):162–8.
10. Heiney SP, Adams SA, Cunningham JE, et al. Subject recruitment for cancer control studies in an adverse environment. Cancer Nurs 2006;29(4):291–9 [quiz: 300–1].
11. Kirchhoff KT, Kehl KA. Recruiting participants in end-of-life research. Am J Hosp Palliat Care 2007;24(6):515–21.
12. Cotter RB, Burke JD, Loeber R, et al. Predictors of contact difficulty and refusal in a longitudinal study. Crim Behav Ment Health 2005;15(2):126–37.
13. Sisk JE, Horowitz CR, Wang JJ, et al. The success of recruiting minorities, women, and elderly into a randomized controlled effectiveness trial. Mt Sinai J Med 2008;75(1):37–43.
14. Alvarez RA, Vasquez E, Mayorga CC, et al. Increasing minority research participation through community organization outreach. West J Nurs Res 2006;28(5):541–60 [discussion: 561–3].
15. Wiegand DL, Norton SA, Baggs JG. Challenges in conducting end-of-life research in critical care. AACN Adv Crit Care 2008;19(2):170–7.
16. Resnick B, Concha B, Burgess JG, et al. Recruitment of older women: lessons learned from the Baltimore Hip Studies. Nurs Res 2003;52(4):270–3.

17. Tansey CM, Matte AL, Needham D, et al. Review of retention strategies in longitudinal studies and application to follow-up of ICU survivors. Intensive Care Med 2007;33(12):2051–7.
18. Robinson KA, Dennison CR, Waynam DM, et al. Systematic review identifies number of strategies important for retaining study participants. J Clin Epidemiol 2007;60(8):757–65.
19. Spilsbury K, Peterick E, Cullum N, et al. The role and potential contribution of clinical research nurses to clinical trials. J Clin Nurs 2008;17(4):549–57.

Practical Issues in Conducting Hospital-based Research

Cheryl A. Lehman, PhD, RN, CNS

KEYWORDS

- Hospital-based research • Hospital research
- Nursing research • Issues in research • Research validity

Hospitals do not lend themselves easily to research. Like any business, hospitals have their own unique focus and their own specific goals. The primary focus of hospitals is patient care, with an emphasis on the goals of timeliness, patient satisfaction, and cost-effectiveness. Hospitals have outside pressure from payors to quickly process patients, beginning with a swift admission and fast work-up, with rapid solution of the patient's problem and a speedy discharge to an appropriate setting. Hospitals are also subject to external pressures and regulations from local, state and federal governments in addition to accrediting and certifying agencies. Hospitals must manage day-to-day pressures, such as staffing, morale, and unforeseen emergencies, as well as long-term pressures, such as patient outcomes and financial income. Hospitals are busy, chaotic places, dealing with everything from patients and families with compliments and complaints, to equipment and supplies with breakages and costs. Hospitals unquestionably have their own peculiar culture with unique priorities unrelated to research.

Although the business of the hospital is patients, research in the hospital setting is important. Clinicians, patients and administrators can all benefit from learning more about the care and practices in hospitals and interventions that could improve outcomes, but the priorities, practices, policies and mores of the hospital can affect the feasibility of performing any type of research in the setting, as well as the reliability and validity of data collected in that setting. Patient, staff, administration and system issues can all impact research in the hospital. Those performing or assisting with research in the hospital setting should be aware of the potential challenges, so that plans can be made to avoid or minimize problems and adjust for planned and unplanned changes in the conduct of their studies.

Acute Nursing Department, The University of Texas Health Science Center at San Antonio, School of Nursing, 7703 Floyd Curl Drive, San Antonio, TX 78229-3900, USA
E-mail address: lehmanc@uthscsa.edu

Perioperative Nursing Clinics 4 (2009) 269–276
doi:10.1016/j.cpen.2009.05.008 **periopnursing.theclinics.com**
1556-7931/09/$ – see front matter

TYPES OF RESEARCH IN THE HOSPITAL

Multiple kinds of research are performed in the hospital setting. Hospital-based research includes patient-focused studies, research about hospital staff and equipment used in the institutions, and investigation into hospital practices and systems. Research can concern the patients on a particular unit or patients of a certain age. Researchers may investigate professionals as diverse as nurses and housekeepers. Speed of access to equipment, equipment reliability and breakdown rates, and equipment accuracy are all potential areas of study. Systems, such as laboratory processes or documentation, also lend themselves to formal study.

The *Journal of Neuroscience Nursing* recently published three reports of hospital-based research concerning patients, nurses, and systems in a single issue. Marie Lasater presented a case study of a patient with an epidural hematoma who received intravascular temperature modulation as an adjunct for secondary brain injury prevention.[1] Marit Silen, Ping Fen Tank, Barbra Wadensten and Gerd Ahlstrom[2] reported a qualitative study of Swedish nurses' experiences of workplace stress and the occurrence of ethical dilemmas in a neurologic setting. Breeda O'Farrell and Guang Yong Zou[3] discussed program evaluation of the implementation of a stroke assessment tool.

Hospital-based research often includes use of the medical record. For instance, a retrospective study could be entirely based on documentation in the medical records, and a prospective study could employ the medical records currently in use on the unit. There could be a mix of paper and electronic records as health care facilities transition to fully electronic records. The researcher may also need to use microfiche or microfilm records.

TYPES OF RESEARCHERS

Researchers who conduct studies in the hospital setting include nurses, physicians, therapists, allied health personnel, administrators, students, faculty, and health services researchers. This list is only illustrative and certainly not exhaustive. Less formal research methods are commonly used by the institution to investigate quality issues, such as pressure ulcer incidence and patient satisfaction. More formal, controlled methods of research, such as experimental designs using randomized assignment to comparison groups and rigorously designed and implemented interventions, are often employed by funded researchers to learn more about a topic and to evaluate interventions.

The researcher may be an "insider" or an "outsider." Either status could affect the success of the study. Insiders may have some advantages because they know more about the culture of the facility and they know more people within the facility. It may be easier for the insider to get permission from administration to conduct research at the facility, have credibility for the research questions being asked and the methods used, and get staff involvement in the study. On the other hand, insiders may believe that they know more about the culture than they actually do; they may make assumptions about the culture, innuendos, behaviors and language that are not true or they may have a lack of objectivity that will negatively affect the study. The insider also may experience blurred lines with staff regarding which role the researcher is playing at any moment: a hospital provider or an objective scientist.[4] Additionally, an insider may have other "baggage" from their own personal history, both professional and social, within the hospital that an outsider would not carry along.

The type of research conducted, as well as the status of the researcher, will affect the feasibility of the study. Patient-focused research may require access to the patients and/or medical records. It may also require involvement of the family and the hospital staff. Also, it undeniably requires approval and support from the administration. Staff-focused research will probably require time from the staff and support from administration. Systems-focused research could require involvement across departments, with a need for staff involvement and administrative support.

CHALLENGES TO HOSPITAL-BASED RESEARCH: THE PATIENT

Ask anyone who works in the hospital: patients are sicker than in years past.[5,6] Patient turnover is also higher giving shorter intervals for study of patients healthy enough to be active research participants. The case manager has become the person responsible for "getting the patient out" as quickly as is safe. This means that the pace of care is hectic: multiple procedures and tests are scheduled closely together with little "down-time." Radiology and other ancillary departments often remain open around the clock to accommodate the need to perform radiographs and tests as efficiently as possible. All of these elements are real or potential obstacles to patient-focused research.

Researchers will often find themselves in competition with care providers, eg, physicians on rounds, nurses providing personal care, therapists scheduling therapy on or off the unit, transporters arriving to transport the patient to another test or procedure, case managers working on discharge planning, chaplains, dietitians, and pharmacists working to assess the patient and plan care. In the teaching hospital, add in a variety of students all wanting access to the patient. Patients, being as a group sicker than in past years, may not feel well enough to participate in a study that requires them to perform or engage in speech or behavioral activity. Patients may be fatigued from multiple procedures and tests, and also may be transferred to another unit or discharged to home without the researcher's knowledge.[7]

Redeker[8] found unique challenges in conducting a hospital-based sleep study in critically ill adults. Fifty percent of sleep occurs in the daylight hours in the critical care setting, necessitating special procedures to monitor sleep in study subjects. Care occurs around the clock in intensive care units (ICUs), and it is not always possible to control environmental stimuli when testing interventions for sleep. Another hospital-based study with older adults revealed that background noise and distractions, present in most hospitals, interfered with data collection.[7] This study also documented numerous interruptions and delays in the study interview process due to physician visits, tests off of the unit, and patient illness.

The hospitalized patient may have physical, cognitive or sensory impairments that affect participation and data quality. Berkman and colleagues[7] found many conditions that interfered with their study of older hospitalized adults. These conditions included: moderate or severe illness (24.1% of participants); delirium (0.8% of participants); physical symptoms (5.5% of participants); hearing disorders (28.8% of participants); and pain, coughing or shortness of breath (12.1% of participants).

CHALLENGES TO HOSPITAL-BASED RESEARCH: THE STAFF

Staff can affect hospital-based research in several different ways. For one, the staff may be the gateway to the patient in patient-focused research. They might identify patients for the researchers, obtained informed consent, administer interventions, or document patient conditions, such as vital signs as a part of the researcher's data collection. Nurses are the logical partners in conducting in-hospital research. Nurses, after all, are at the hospital 24 hours a day, 7 days per week. The researcher, however, may find it difficult to engage nurses for a number of reasons, including staff knowledge, staffing patterns, staff motivation, vacations, holidays, and sick call.

Staff knowledge of the research process is important if they are to be actively involved. Nursing staff is made up of many levels with many different educational backgrounds and not all nurses receive research training. Nursing assistants provide the majority of direct patient care. They have likely had no training in research, and minimal training in medical topics. Licensed Vocational Nurses (LVNs) have had one year of training, are licensed by the state, and are not likely to have any research training. They are employed in differing roles, ranging from medication administration to employing the primary care model of care delivery. Registered nurses are educated at the diploma, ADN and BSN levels, with 2–4 years of higher education. Not all have received training in research and not all have been exposed to research in practice or in other ways, such as journals or conferences. Temporary and traveling nurses are not unusual in many settings. The varied level of nurses' exposure to research, with little or no exposure in their own education and practice being predominant, makes it sometimes difficult to engage them in active research roles in hospitals. This situation may lead to inconsistencies across nurses engaged in such roles.

Nursing staff, on any particular shift, may have a patient load with high acuity that requires 100% of their time. They may be short-staffed because of call-ins, or may have had some staff pulled to other units. There may be unforeseen emergencies that consume their time. System issues may make their job even harder, as they try to locate supplies and medications that are missing. The staff may not be a fully functioning team, and they may have interpersonal issues that can affect the research. Nursing staff often rotate shifts, have days off, and take vacations. The researcher might train the staff on one unit to participate in a study, only to encounter times where per-diem nurses are filling in for permanent staff members who are on vacation. Floating staff may compromise the integrity of a study if they floated from a unit involved in another arm of the same study. Staff who were off during training for the study, or who are new to the unit, may affect the study without knowing. Again, all these factors have potential to reduce nurses' engagement in roles supportive of research projects and may lead to inconsistencies within the components of a given study.

Staff motivation is an issue in research. Motivation problems can affect every aspect of research conducted in the hospital. Staff may even be biased against research, and subtly work to sabotage a particular study or researcher. They may see the duties related to the study as extra work, as not important, as ridiculous, or as interfering with unit function.

There is also competition with department needs. Nursing units and departments require their staff to work on projects other than patient care in their free time. So staff may be conducting quality studies on their units, with chart reviews and observation of care. They may be preparing for accreditation or certification of their workplace from a body like the state Department of Health, The Joint Commission, or Magnet reviewers. They may be required to participate in self-governance activities away from the unit. They may simply not be available to the researcher, especially if the researcher is seen as using up their valuable time.

Staff trust may affect the research study in the hospital setting.[4] Staff may feel that there is a hidden agenda, that the researcher is going to expose their shortcomings, or that the researcher will benefit but that they will not. If staff members are collecting data for the researcher, this situation could affect accuracy or completeness of data. If staff are the subjects of the study, this could affect the reliability or validity of results obtained. "Images and myths" of the staff can also affect a research study. Staff in one nursing home study strongly believed that patients with dementia should receive blenderized food. Although the researchers taught the staff differently, staff continued to blenderize food for patients not being fed directly by the researchers.

This action on the part of the staff meant that the researchers were unable to eliminate competing hypotheses in the interpretation of their results.[9]

Phillips and Van Ort[9] further realized the strong influence of staff on the success of their study. Staff refused to allow one of the participants in the study to come to the dining room for meals, requiring a change in research protocol for this single patient. This situation affected the study's internal validity, particularly because there was a small pool of patients from which to draw participants and thus the inclusion of this participant was important to the study. These researchers noted that the power dynamics of the facility in which they conducted their study were a major factor in their ability to conduct the study. Research interventions were not performed unless the researchers were physically present. Nonprofessional staff members were able to sabotage the filming stage of the study, by rearranging their meal times or making certain patients unavailable for filming.

Primary care providers or attending physicians can present another challenge. There may be a feeling of territoriality, eg, "This is my patient, not yours." A physician might not allow a patient to consent to participate in a study if the topic is a sensitive one. Froman and Owen,[10] when studying attitudes and use of advance directives of patients hospitalized 3 days or more, found one physician would not allow any of his patients to participate because he believed they needed no advance directives because they "were not going to die." (Froman, personal communication, January 10, 2009). Again, the goals of the provider and researcher may differ: the provider's duty is to clinically manage the patient while attending to fiscal responsibilities and other pressures associated with the patient's care.

CHALLENGES TO HOSPITAL-BASED RESEARCH: THE ENVIRONMENT

Privacy and confidentiality are difficult to ensure in the hospital setting, which can affect the research. Not all patients are in private rooms, and not all nursing units have private conference rooms with doors that are available to the researcher to close for privacy or to lock to secure data. Hancock, Chenoweth and Chang[11] found that patients would give different responses to surveys when the nurse was present. It was postulated that the patients may have been afraid of criticizing nursing care within nurses' hearing because of a sense of vulnerability. HIPAA regulations add another layer of complexity to the privacy, confidentiality and data management issues.

Documentation is frequently an issue in hospital-based research. The researcher will need to comply with facility policy regarding access to the electronic medical records. As well as having permission from the institutional review board, the researcher may have to traverse a bureaucracy of forms, permissions and training before gaining access to the electronic medical record. Paper records also present challenges; illegible writing and missing pages are common. For retrospective studies, the researcher must deal with a formal medical records department and comply with facility rules regarding access to records. Records that have been formally filed may be stored at other sites, and requests for records, must often be made several days or even weeks in advance.

The legal environment of the hospital may affect the feasibility of conducting research at a specific facility. The researcher may be asked to be formally credentialed at the institution, a process that can take several months. Facilities may require approval from internal institutional review boards as well as the review board of the researcher's employer, if the researcher is not an employee at the institution. Administrative approval up and down the chain of command may be required, in addition to approval by individual departments affected by the study.

Studies conducted with patients in a single facility or unit may not be generalizable (externally valid) because of the homogeneous characteristics of patients in the institution, the unique facility environment, and concurrent treatments that the patient may be receiving.[8] External validity may also be compromised by lack of randomized or representative samples or failure to fully describe the characteristics of the setting.[8] As previously mentioned, internal validity may also be compromised because of the chaotic hospital environment (field noise), making it difficult to guarantee that the experimental treatment is consistently applied or was responsible for the observed effects, rather than uncontrolled and unexpected factors.[8]

OVERCOMING THE CHALLENGES OF THE HOSPITAL SETTING: THE PATIENT

A researcher should be accommodating and flexible in their approach to the situation on the nursing unit, when involved in patient-focused studies. Patients and staff have duties related to the patient's admission and care, and the patient's care is the primary focus of the hospital setting. A researcher may have to return to the unit several times before being connected with the participant.[11] A researcher should maintain flexibility in locating patients for recruitment, as the natural progression of the patient in the hospital system dictates the current trend toward faster discharges and transfers out of the hospital. This means that a researcher may need to eliminate participants from a study because of attrition that cannot be controlled.[11]

Researchers should avoid recruitment of patients during mealtimes, immediately after therapy or treatments, or immediately after unforeseen incidents, such as a fall.[11] Researchers should include time in their plan for follow-up for busy patients. Staff needs to complete their work with the patient, and allow the patient to participate in hospital activities and tests. It may be difficult and frustrating to defer research, but it is important to remember that the patient is in the hospital for medical treatment.

Researchers should be aware of the burden the study presents to the participants, and consider streamlining interviews and interventions. Pretesting interviews can help to better estimate the time it takes to complete. Researchers should express appreciation and respect for the patient's time, as well as recognize symptomatic distress, patient agitation, or other situations where they might best postpone time with the participant.[7]

OVERCOMING THE CHALLENGES OF THE HOSPITAL SETTING: THE STAFF

Staff may be partners or participants in hospital-based research. Whatever their role, it is important to engage them from the beginning of the study. Researchers should become familiar with current issues on the unit that may affect a study and determine how to adjust the study accordingly to minimize adverse effects on the data. One should respect the staff's workload and commit to minimizing their burden. A researcher might consider helping with part of their workload to facilitate adherence to their own role in the study.[12] Resarchers can spend time with staff on all shifts, getting to know their routines and culture.[13]

A research study should ensure clarity on who has responsibility for study procedures: enrollment, informed consent, interventions, data collection. All involved should be aware of the study protocol and those involved should be adequately trained, realizing that the amount of training will vary depending upon the people being trained.[14]

Staff contributions should be recognized. This recognition can be done in multiple ways, including: tangible rewards of food or money; recognition in print in local newspapers or in association with a manuscript produced from the study; or with a frequent and simple "thank you." One should consider involving the staff in the dissemination of results.[12] The results of the study and its findings should be shared with the staff. Omission of that final step is certain to have negative results if researchers wish to return to the same hospital setting for subsequent research studies.

The staff may have practices and habits that may not be congruent with a particular research study, and that these practices and habits may be difficult to change and maintain. Inclusion of staff from the beginning in planning the study, and provision of adequate training and oversight can help minimize staff bias.

There are multiple sources of power in the hospital. Although researchers may gain administrative support, unless the staff most proximate to the study support it, data may be compromised. Sources of formal and informal power should be identified, and strategies planned to gain the support of both formal and informal leaders. Staff and administrators should be included in planning study procedures.[13]

It is important to stress how the research study can help those in the hospital setting. Will it potentially benefit the patient, nurse or administrator? Will it make patients better, ease nurses' workload, or contain costs? Will it aid in retention of nurses, increase nurses' safety, or document an effective intervention? Engaging the staff by garnering enthusiasm for the aims of the study will facilitate a smoother process. The staff should be kept informed and involved through communication and contact.[9]

It may be necessary to allow for staff attrition and ever-changing staff. Depending upon the depth of staff involvement in a particular study, there should be a plan for compensating for rotating staff members. Also, a plan for meeting with staff should be developed. If the staff are participants, researchers may need to introduce and discuss the study, especially "what's in it for them." If they are partners in the study, researchers should decide how much training the staff will need and how quality will be maintained.

OVERCOMING THE CHALLENGES OF THE HOSPITAL SETTING: THE ENVIRONMENT

Blinding is often not feasible in the complex and chaotic health care setting, and assumptions that "usual care" is static may be mistaken. Care delivered as "usual care" may in fact change over time or may be different between units or clinicians.[15,16] Researchers should anticipate changes in standards of care.[16]

Researchers should become familiar with their research environment posing questions such as "will noise and chaos interfere with data collection? Can we ensure confidentiality?" Researchers may need to negotiate to use private conference rooms or offices for interviews. Some facilities may have formal reservation systems to regulate access to private spaces.

Researchers should learn the policies of the institution in regard to credentialing, access to electronic records and access to paper records. One should ask the medical records personnel how long it will take to obtain a previously filed record, and what are the rules for viewing it. Also, researchers should investigate the policy on conducting research in this institution, the institutional review board rules, and any limitations that may be encountered concerning access to patients, staff or records.

Researchers should consult with the admission office, the care manager, and the nursing staff on ways to track patients throughout the admission. This strategy will depend on the structure of the study, but researchers may need to devise methods of staying informed of the anticipated and actual discharge date.

SUMMARY

Research in the hospital setting is challenging but important, necessary and "doable." It is in vivo research with all the associated benefits and real obstacles. Studies can be facilitated through inclusion of hospital administrators and staff from the early planning stages. The researcher must be aware of potential threats to the reliability and validity of data, and take steps to minimize these threats. Although it may be difficult to overcome the challenges of conducting research in the hospital setting, the more the researcher learns about the setting, the easier it will be. The astute and responsible researcher will recognize the limitations of the study conducted in the hospital setting, and will communicate these limitations during the dissemination of results. Researchers are encouraged to conduct studies within the hospital setting to the benefit of patients, staff, and administrators.

REFERENCES

1. Lasater M. Intravascular temperature modulation as an adjunct to secondary brain injury prevention in a patient with an epidural hematoma. J Neurosci Nurs 2008;40:198–200.
2. Silen M, Tang PF, Wadensten B, et al. Workplace distress and ethical dilemmas in neuroscience nursing. J Neurosci Nurs 2008;40:222–31.
3. O'Farrell B, Zou GY. Implementation of the Canadian neurological scale on an acute care neuroscience unit: a program evaluation. J Neurosci Nurs 2008;40:201–11.
4. Asselin MF. Insider research: issues to consider when doing qualitative research in your own setting. J Nurses Staff Dev 2003;19:99–103.
5. Thomson Reuters, 2007. Hospitals improve survival rates while treating sicker patients. Available at: http://employer.thomsonhealthcare.com/News/view/?id=1265. Accessed January 8, 2009.
6. Welton JM. 2007. Mandatory hospital nurse to patient staffing ratios: time to take a different approach. Online J Issues Nurs. Available at: http://www.nursingworld.org/MainMenuCategories/ANAMarketplace/ANAPeriodicals/OJIN/TableofContents/Volume122007/No3Sept07/andatoryNursetoPatientRatios.aspx. Accessed January 8, 2009.
7. Berkman CS, Leipzig RM, Greenberg SA, et al. Methodologic issues in conducting research on hospitalized older people. J Am Geriatr Soc 2001;49:172–8.
8. Redeker NS. Challenges and opportunities associated with studying sleep in critically ill adults. AACN Adv Crit Care 2008;19:178–85.
9. Phillips LR, Van Ort S. Issues in conducting intervention research in long-term care settings. Nurs Outlook 1995;43:249–53.
10. Froman RD, Owen SV. Randomized study of stability and change in patients' advance directives. Res Nurs Health 2005;28:398–407.
11. Hancock K, Chenoweth L, Chang E. Challenges in conducting research with acutely hospitalized older adults. Nurs Health Sci 2003;5:253–9.
12. Chan GK, Houweling L, Leet T, et al. Conducting research in the emergency department: Respect nurses' workload and recognize their contribution. J Emerg Nurs 2000;26:626–7.
13. Maas ML, Kelley LS, Park M, et al. Issues in conducting research in nursing homes. West J Nurs Res 2002;24:373–89.
14. Nelson P, Adamson A, Moore H. Conducting randomized controlled trials in primary care: lessons learned from an obesity management trial. Br J Gen Pract 2006;56:674–9.
15. Guihan M, Garber SL, Bombardier CH, et al. Lessons learned while conducting research on prevention of pressure ulcers in veterans with spinal cord injury. Arch Phys Med Rehabil 2007;88:858–61.
16. Vanderploeg RD, Collins RC, Sigford B, et al. Practical and theoretical considerations in designing rehabilitation trials: the DVBIC cognitive-didactic versus functional-experiential treatment study experience. J Head Trauma Rehabil 2006;21:179–93.

Bridging the Gap Between Research and Clinical Practice

Sharon L. Lewis, RN, PhD, FAAN[a,b,*]

KEYWORDS

- Research barriers • Research facilitators
- Nursing research • Clinical practice
- Evidenced-based practice • Nursing practice

Hilda, a nurse with 10 years of experience, is teaching a patient with a healing well-granulated wound to irrigate it every day with hydrogen peroxide. Cory, a new nurse who is in the patient's room, is listening to this conversation. She knows that what Hilda is teaching is not correct but is reluctant to say anything. A few hours later, Cory discusses the patient with Hilda and mentions that peroxide treatment is not appropriate for this patient's wound. Hilda replies, "This is the way we always do it and I want to make sure that the wound is really clean." Cory, faced with a dilemma, does not know whether she should alienate Hilda or show her the research findings that document the best practices for wound care.

Do we want patients to have health care based on the latest and best knowledge or should they be treated with traditional and ritualistic methods? The best clinical practices are based on research. The primary purposes of nursing research are (1) to expand the knowledge base for nursing practice and (2) to improve the quality of patient care (**Fig. 1**). In addition to improving patient care, nursing research can reduce health care costs.[1] For this to happen, relevant research needs to be incorporated into clinical practice. Research is of little value unless it is used; however, research findings are not being implemented even when there is evidence that integration of these findings would produce more effective patient outcomes and better clinical practice.[2] Patients suffer unfortunate consequences when advances in research are not incorporated into practice.[3–5]

For many years it has been recognized that a gap exists between what is known (based on research) and what is done in clinical practice. At least 30% to 40% of

[a] Schools of Nursing and Medicine, University of Texas Health Science Center at San Antonio, San Antonio, TX, USA
[b] GRECC 182, South Texas Veterans Health Care System, 7400 Merton Minter Boulevard, San Antonio, TX 78229, USA
* GRECC 182, South Texas Veterans Health Care System, 7400 Merton Minter Boulevard, San Antonio, TX 78229.
E-mail address: lewissl@uthscsa.edu

Perioperative Nursing Clinics 4 (2009) 277–286
doi:10.1016/j.cpen.2009.05.004 periopnursing.theclinics.com
1556-7931/09/$ – see front matter

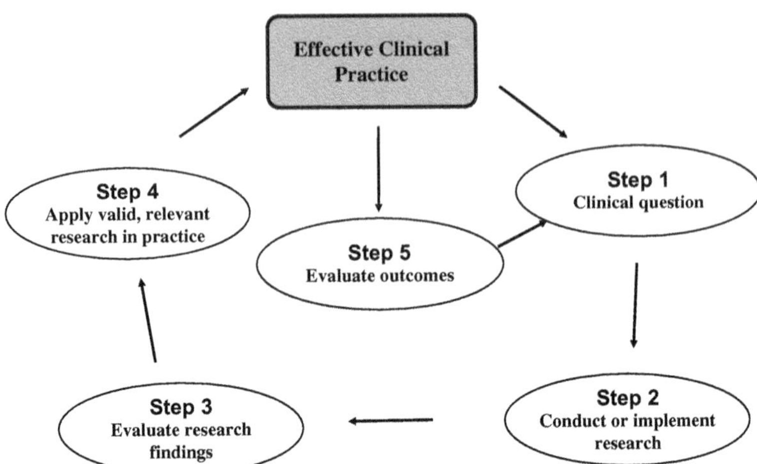

Fig. 1. Effective clinical practice results from identifying questions or issues of concern in clinical practice. Research is then conducted or existing research findings are implemented. Research findings are evaluated and then relevant findings are applied to clinical practice.

patients do not receive care based on current scientific evidence, and 20% or more of the care provided is not needed or potentially harmful to patients.[6] In addition, a time lag from 8 to 30 years exists between the availability of research evidence and its application to practice.[7,8]

When attitudes and beliefs about research are explored, nurses have an overwhelming positive attitude about research. They also believe that nursing practice should be based on research;[9,10] however, a positive attitude alone will not change practice. It is imperative that nursing develops a research-based practice. Nurses need to use research findings to develop enhanced assessment skills, revise policies and procedures, and develop effective interventions so that research findings will translate to improved patient outcomes. The primary purposes of this article are (1) to identify barriers to using research in clinical practice and (2) to discuss effective ways to facilitate integration of research findings in clinical practice.

BARRIERS TO USING RESEARCH IN CLINICAL PRACTICE

Barriers to using research in clinical practice can be divided into organizational and nurse barriers (**Table 1**).

Organizational Barriers

Organizational barriers are those that occur in the work setting. Many studies have identified organizational barriers as the most frequent barriers to research implementation.[10–15] The two key organizational barriers are (1) nurses' lack of time to read research or implement research-based practice and (2) lack of nursing authority to change practice. Other organizational barriers are listed in **Table 1**.

Nurse Barriers

Nurse barriers are related to the nurse and are personal barriers (see **Table 1**). Many nurses do not have the research training and skill sets to critically read and evaluate

Table 1
Most common barriers to using research in clinical practice

Organizational	Nurse
Inadequate time to read research or evidence-based practice articles	Not capable of/difficulty with critically reading and evaluating research articles
Insufficient time at job to implement research or new ideas	Difficulty accessing or unaware of research in clinical area of interest
Feeling powerless or lacking authority to change procedures/practices related to patient care	Resistance to change, unwilling/uninterested to change or try new ideas
Lack of support from administration and physicians to conduct or implement research	Lacking research skills to conduct or implement research
Nursing staff are not supportive of conducting or implementing research	Nurse isolated from knowledgeable colleagues

research articles. Many nurses have not had research or statistics classes because they were not provided in their educational courses. Lack of research skills results in an inability or lack of confidence in conducting or implementing research. If nurses do not understand research, they cannot apply it to practice.

The longer nurses practice, the simpler it is to do what is easier or what is familiar to them. Hilda irrigated the wound with peroxide because she had always done it this way. She did not take into consideration what type of wound it was or what research evidence indicates as the best practice. Hilda also was resistant to change even when Cory suggested that there may a more effective way to treat the wound.

FACILITATORS FOR USING RESEARCH IN CLINICAL PRACTICE

To facilitate the use of research in clinical practice, organizations and individual nurses need to get involved to improve patient outcomes (**Table 2**). One of the first steps in facilitating research is to identify the barriers in implementing research. An effective tool to use is the BARRIERS Scale.[16] This scale measures perceptions of barriers regarding the nurse, the setting, the research, and the presentation of research. Results of studies that have used this scale have been reviewed.[17–19]

After the barriers are identified, strategies can be developed to overcome these barriers. Insight into the obstacles that exist in delivering evidence-based care will frequently pave the way for a plan that yields success and improves patient outcomes.

Organizational Facilitation

Creating a culture in which research and evidence-based practice are valued and expected is probably the most critical strategy for organizational facilitation. As part of this effort, administrative support and encouragement are key elements for success (see **Table 2**). Administrators are responsible for creating an environment that fosters and promotes the use of research in practice. Because of their ability to shape the practice environment, administrators have a pivotal role in promoting research-based practice and are in a primary position to affect the dissemination and use of research findings.[20]

Fink and colleagues[21] found that lack of time, mentorship, and support from supervisors were barriers to research implementation that could be improved by a commitment from the organization. They emphasized that creating an organizational climate

Table 2
Most effective facilitators for using research in clinical practice

Organizational	Nurse
Incorporate research into the goals/ mission of the organization	Find research articles that are relevant to clinical practice
Create an organizational climate of intellectual curiosity that values the use of research	Develop journal club where clinical problems are presented and research articles discussed
Incorporate research in nurses' job descriptions and responsibilities	Participate in informal special interest research groups
Reward nurses who conduct research or implement research-based protocols	Attend and participate in formal research classes and inservice education to increase research knowledge
Enhance organization support for understanding research (eg, pay for nurses to attend research symposium or research courses, provide staff development activities on research reading and critique)	Attend research symposia or conferences Participate in research rounds
Implement research grand rounds or other clinical research presentations by nurses	Develop formal or informal collaboration with nurse faculty colleagues
Provide opportunities for nurses to participate in clinically focused, relevant research (eg, develop interdisciplinary research teams)	Find nurses with research skills to serve as role models and mentors
Provide inservice education on how to conduct library searches on clinical topics of interest to staff	Establish a formal research committee
	Develop newsletter that highlights research findings
	Use bulletin board to highlight research findings
	Participate in clinically focused, relevant research

that values research use and supports nurses to participate in such activities is crucial to the organization's success.

Administrators can communicate support for research through incorporating use of research in job descriptions and performance appraisal criteria. The administration needs to allocate the funds and key resources, such as making journals available, having online access to journals and Web sites, providing necessary staff development activities to foster skill in reading and evaluating research, allowing the staff time to read and participate in discussion of research articles, developing policy and procedures or protocols to implement changes in practice, and finding a way to recognize and reward successful use of research in practice. The more opportunities nurses have to read and discuss research, the more likely they are to implement research in practice.

Allocating a percentage of time for advanced practice nurses (APNs) to facilitate research is another possible strategy that can be used. These APNs can (1) search the literature for answers to clinical questions, (2) organize and present research rounds, and (3) provide the leadership for a journal club.

Focus groups (ie, group discussions that facilitate open communication) can be conducted to determine nurses' knowledge, attitudes, and beliefs about research and challenges in implementing evidence-based care. The results of these groups provide essential information for nursing staff and administrators on how to implement effective strategies.

Establishing a department of nursing research indicates the organization's commitment to research. An expert nurse researcher can help to mentor, support, and motivate novice researchers and engage them in various parts of the research process (see later discussion on models).

The use of research and evidence-based practice is a key component of obtaining Magnet status which hospitals seek to secure. The Magnet Recognition Program was developed by the American Nurses Credentialing Center (ANCC) to recognize health care organizations that provide nursing excellence.[22,23] Magnet status is an award given by the ANCC, an affiliate of the American Nurses Association, to hospitals that satisfy a set of criteria designed to measure the strength and quality of their nursing. A Magnet hospital is one where nursing delivers excellent patient outcomes, nurses have a high level of job satisfaction, and there is a low staff nurse turnover rate. Magnet status also indicates that nursing is involved in shaping research-based nursing practice and nurses are rewarded for advancing nursing practice. For those hospitals seeking to obtain or maintain Magnet status, implementing research and evidence-based practice is essential.

Nurses need time away from the responsibilities of bedside care, autonomy over their practice, education in finding and assessing research, access to research, and mentorship to guide them through the implementation process and didactic learning.[12] Communicating support for research involves the creation of an organizational culture that values and uses research and one in which research questions are welcomed and nursing care is systematically evaluated. If nurses are allowed to question current clinical practices, such questioning will become the expectation will rather than the exception. When nurses believe that the environment is conducive to questioning current practice and searching for more effective practice, they believe they have the authority to change practice using research.

Nurse Facilitation

Regardless of the organization's efforts, research-based practice will not become a reality until the clinical nurse embraces the idea that research is important. Nurses need to be inquisitive. They must continually ask questions. Is this the most effective way to provide care? Does current research support what we do? Are these practices consistent with the guidelines established by professional nurse organizations or national organizations such as the Centers for Disease Control and Prevention?

Nurses should be encouraged to update their research skills through seeking advanced education and taking formal research courses. Local schools of nursing can provide education about research and how to use it. Nurses should attend conferences in their clinical area of interest as practice updates and research findings are presented.

Although nurses may read research articles and value research, they may need additional assistance in implementing these research findings in their practice setting. One strategy that can be effective is journal clubs. These clubs involve a group of nurses who are willing to commit to a regularly scheduled forum in which they review and discuss research articles, systematic reviews, or evidence-based protocols. A journal club is a non-threatening setting where ideas and thought-provoking questions can be freely exchanged and discussed. Another idea is to personalize the scenario and ask, "What kind of wound care would you want if...?" Personalizing these scenarios can stimulate motivation to investigate best practices described in the literature and change practice.

A journal club topic on wound care may help Hilda realize that there are other ways to care for wounds besides using peroxide. Had Hilda ever questioned her wound care practices? Did she realize that there are different wound therapies based on the type of wound or is she comfortable with the "because we have always done it this way" approach? Does she realize that her wound care is actually harming the patient? Because hydrogen peroxide can damage the new epithelium of healing tissue, it should never be used in a clean granulating wound.

Nurses need to get involved as members of research teams. A study by Bostrum and Suter[9] concluded that nurse involvement in research-related activities (eg, data collection) is the best predictor of the use of research findings in clinical practice.

Another facilitative technique is research rounds. Research rounds are regularly scheduled forums. They can take the format of having an individual with expertise in a substantive area agree to search for, critique, and appraise the evidence to answer a compelling clinical question, such as "What is the most effective care for wounds?" They may also be used to have nurses present their own research ideas or research studies.

Nurses who read research improve their critical thinking and are motivated to expand the ways in which they view patient situations, assess problems, and plan care.[21] Perceptions of themselves as professionals are enhanced, and their work becomes more interesting and fulfilling.[20]

EFFECTIVE MODELS FOR REMOVING BARRIERS AND IMPLEMENTING RESEARCH

University of New Mexico Hospital

To promote nursing research, the University of New Mexico Hospital (UNMH) in Albuquerque, New Mexico, hired a Director of Clinical Nursing Research. In this role Dr. Kathy Lopez-Bushnell helps to mentor and facilitate research within the clinical practice setting. Over the past 10 years this position has improved the conducting and implementation of research and helped nurses put evidence-based practice into action.[24] Some of the strategies that have been used at UNMH to promote research within the practice setting are described in **Table 3**.

Nurses at the staff and management levels have gotten involved in research. These nurses recognize that research improves patient care. An atmosphere and milieu of excitement about research permeates the hospital. Over 50 applications for nursing research have been submitted for institutional review board approval from nurses at the hospital. Many nurses have given research presentations regionally and nationally. Manuscripts have been submitted for publication, and some have already been published. Grants have been written and funded.

A key to the success at UNMH has been administrative support. The nurses have been provided with a clinical nurse scientist as a mentor and motivator. They have also been provided with secretarial, library, technical, and statistical support. Some nurses have been provided with release time to conduct research; however, research still requires that the nurses devote much of their personal time to conducting and implementing research.

University Hospital at San Antonio

Ventilator-associated pneumonia (VAP) is the leading cause of morbidity and mortality in intensive care units (ICUs).[25] ICU nurses at the University Hospital in San Antonio,

Table 3
Strategies used to promote research at the University of New Mexico Hospital

Strategy	Description
Nursing research council	Established to determine the hospital's research foci and recruit interested nurses Meets once/month
Research rounds	Similar to grand rounds but focuses on nursing research at the hospital Meets once/month Presentations done by various nurses involved in research Continuing education credits available for participants
Survey on barriers to use of research	Survey of nurses conducted to determine barriers to using research Results presented at research rounds
Nursing research course for nurse leaders	Course designed for nurse leaders Nurses receive university credit as well as continuing education credits Provides impetus for nurses to start their own research projects
Internship program	12-month program that teaches staff nurses the basics of research, including how to conduct research and implement research findings
State nursing research conference	Jointly planned between UNMH nurses and College of Nursing faculty Provides opportunities for hospital nurses to present research findings
Nursing residence program	New graduates who are hired can chose to participate in a 2-year program that provides a mentor for clinical expertise, supervised clinical rotations to units of choice, and 15 university graduate credit hours that include research experience After completion, able to facilitate research projects with designated time in their schedules
Staff nurses involved in research	Each staff nurse encouraged to start or participate in a research study

Texas, were concerned about the rates of VAP. The nurses also wondered if the oral care of intubated patients met national professional standards suggested by the American Association of Critical Care Nurses and other sources.

Although the nurses believed that oral care was an important aspect of nursing care for these patients, there were no written protocols for oral comfort and hygiene measures for intubated patients. This lack of protocols led the group to ask the following questions: Can oral care measures reduce the incidence of VAP? What specific oral care measures are indicated for patients receiving mechanical ventilation? Which are the most effective? What are effective education activities for teaching staff about oral assessment or oral care?

The need to address these questions led nurse leaders from the hospital and faculty from the affiliated School of Nursing at the University of Texas Health Science Center to create a structured research educational program for the ICU nurses. The goal of the educational program was to enhance the staff nurses' research self-efficacy and develop a spirit of discovery. In fact, the learning groups were called Discovery Groups.

The educational, six-session Critical Reading of Research Publications Plus (CRRP-P) course offered to 17 ICU nurses was developed by Dr. Carol Reineck, a faculty member at the School of Nursing. Evelyn Swenson-Britt, Clinical Research Director for the hospital, added a seventh session on library search skills, bringing in a medical librarian for the program. Each nurse participant received a manual that contained the six lessons from the CRRP along with data-based articles selected from the literature review that exemplified the material being taught. The 6-week sessions included:

Week 1: Introduction of the Research Article
Week 2: Design and Sample
Week 3: Methods-Data Collection Plan and Instruments
Week 4: Interpretation of Descriptive Statistics
Week 5: Interpretation of Inferential Statistics
Week 6: Discussion, Conclusions, Recommendations

With continued support, nine of the nurses from this group developed an oral care survey, completed a protocol for the survey, obtained permission from the institutional review board, and administered the survey on their units. They also used the data to work on a second protocol developing an oral care assessment and training initiative in a collaborative effort with the dental school.

The course in reading research increased the confidence of practicing nurses to use research. This model shows promise for increasing research implementation and improving patient outcomes. Formal research mentoring by doctorally prepared nurses is an educational strategy that can help practicing nurses acquire essential research understanding, generating excitement for understanding and implementing evidence-based practice.

SUMMARY

In today's age of rapidly expanding medical and nursing knowledge and advanced technology, research-based nursing practice is essential. Research provides the scientific foundation to direct nursing practice toward the delivery of high-quality, cost-effective patient care; however, research is not implemented even when nurses know it will improve patient outcomes. Successful bridging of the gap between research and practice will ensure that patients receive the best care. When barriers are specifically identified, appropriate interventions can be planned and implemented to facilitate research integration into clinical practice.

Two successful strategies used by institutions have been described. This issue of *Perioperative Nursing Clinics* can also offer the foundation for the development of a third approach. As described in the introduction to this issue, the articles contained provide a basic primer of the essentials for reading and critiquing research. Individual or group use of the content in this issue can assist clinically based nurses in breaking down some of the barriers to applying research in the practice setting.

REFERENCES

1. Aiken LH, Clarke SP, Sloane DM. Hospital restructuring: does it adversely affect care and outcomes? J Nurs Adm 2000;30(10):457–65.
2. Heater B, Becker A, Olson R. Nursing interventions and patient outcomes: a meta-analysis of studies. Nurs Res 1988;37:303–7.

3. Dufault M. A collaborative model for research development and utilization: process, structure, and outcomes. J Nurs Staff Dev 1995;11(3):139–44.
4. Ehrenberg A, Estabrooks CA. Spotlight on research: why using research matters. J Wound Ostomy Continence Nurs 2004;31(2):62–4.
5. Wallin L, Estabrooks CA, Midodzi WK, et al. Development and validation of a derived measure of research utilization by nurses. Nurs Res 2006;55(3):149–60.
6. Grol R, Grimshaw J. From best evidence to best practice: effective implementation of change. Lancet 2003;362:1225–30.
7. Bostrom J, Wise L. Closing the gap between research and practice. J Nurs Adm 1994;24(5):22–7.
8. Landrum BJ. Marketing innovations to nurse. Part 1. How people adopt innovations. J Wound Ostomy Continence Nurs 1998;25:194–9.
9. Bostrom J, Suter WN. Research utilization: making the link to practice. J Nurs Staff Dev 1993;9:28–34.
10. Lewis SL, Prowant BF, Cooper CL, et al. Nephrology nurses' perception of barriers and facilitators to using research in practice. ANNA J 1998;25:397–406.
11. Boström AM, Nilsson Kajermo K, Nordström G, et al. Barriers to research utilization and research use among registered nurses working in the care of older people: does the BARRIERS scale discriminate between research users and non-research users on perceptions of barriers? Implement Sci 2008;3(24). doi: 10.1186/1748-5908-3-24. Available at: http://www.implementationscience.com/content/3/1/24. Accessed February 3, 2009.
12. Brown CE, Wickline MA, Ecoff L, et al. Nursing practice, knowledge, attitudes and perceived barriers to evidence-based practice at an academic medical center. J Adv Nurs 2009;65(2):371–81.
13. Parahoo K. Barriers to, and facilitators of, research utilization among nurses in Northern Ireland. J Adv Nurs 2000;31(1):89–98.
14. Pettengill MM, Gillies DA, Clark CC. Factors encouraging and discouraging the use of nursing research findings. J Nurs Scholarsh 1994;26:143–7.
15. Retsas A. Barriers to using research evidence in nursing practice. J Adv Nurs 2000;31(3):599–606.
16. Funk SG, Champagne MT, Wiese RA, et al. Barriers: the barriers to research utilization scale. Appl Nurs Res 1991;4:39–45.
17. Bosch M, van der Weijden T, Wensing M, et al. Tailoring quality improvement interventions to identified barriers: a multiple case analysis. J Eval Clin Pract 2007;3(2):161–8.
18. Hutchinson AM, Johnston L. Beyond the BARRIERS scale: commonly reported barriers to research use. J Nurs Adm 2006;36(4):189–99.
19. Shaw B, Cheater F, Baker R, et al. Tailored interventions to overcome identified barriers to change: effects on professional practice and health care outcomes. Cochrane Database Syst Rev 2005;(3):CD005470. Available at: http://www.thecochranelibrary.com. Accessed February 10, 2009.
20. Goode C, Bulechek GM. Research utilization: an organizational process that enhances quality of care. Journal of Nursing Care Quality 1992;Suppl:27–35.
21. Fink R, Thompson CJ, Bonnes D. Overcoming barriers and promoting the use of research in practice. J Nurs Adm 2005;35(3):121–9.
22. American Nurses Credentialing Center 2009. Maryland: Subsidiary of the American Nurses Association. Available at: http://www.nursecredentialing.org/Magnet/ProgramOverview.aspx. Accessed June 10, 2009.
23. The Center for Nursing Advocacy 2003–2008. What is magnet status and how's the whole thing going? Takoma Park (MD): The Center for Nursing

Advocacy. Available at: http://nursingadvocacy.org/faq/magnet.html. Accessed February 10, 2009.
24. Lopez-Bushnell K. Get research-ready. Nurs Manage 2002;33(11):41–4.
25. Mayhall CG. Ventilator-associated pneumonia or not? Contemporary diagnosis In: CDC, editor. Emerging infectious diseases. [Special Issue}. Atlanta (GA): CDC; 2001;7(2). p. 200–4.

Beyond Translated Consents: Culturally Competent Research

Lyda C. Arévalo-Flechas, RN, PhD[a,b,*]

KEYWORDS

- Culturally competent research • Cultural proficiency
- Health disparities • Translation methodology • Meaning

Racial and ethnic minorities, now roughly one third of the US population, are expected to become the majority in 2042, with the nation projected to be 54% minority by 2050.[1] The US population at large enjoyed longer lives and improved health during the latter part of the twentieth century,[2] whereas racial and ethnic minorities, who at the time represented 25% of the population, experienced striking health disparities including a shorter life expectancy, higher rates of cancer, diabetes, stroke, heart disease, substance abuse, and infant mortality, and a lower birth weight than the then majority white population.[2] These disparities have been well documented by the Institute of Medicine.[3] Mitigation of health disparities can be achieved, in part, by the delivery of culturally competent health care. The quest for the knowledge necessary to achieve culturally competent care starts with the inclusion of racial and ethnic minorities in research studies that are culturally competent. If research studies lack cultural competency, all that is being accomplished is an illusion of inclusion.

WHAT IS CULTURAL COMPETENCE?

In 2001, the Office of Minority Health of the US Department of Health and Human Services published the National Standards for Culturally and Linguistically Appropriate

---

This work was supported by The John A. Hartford Foundation Building Academic Geriatric Nursing Capacity Program.

[a] Department of Acute Nursing Care, The University of Texas Health Science Center, San Antonio School of Nursing, 7703 Floyd Curl Drive, Mail Code 7975, San Antonio, TX 78229, USA

[b] The John A. Hartford Foundation, Building Academic Geriatric Nursing Capacity Program, Claire M. Fagin Fellowship, American Academy of Nursing Coordinating Center, 888 17th Street, NW Suite 800, Washington, DC 20006, USA

* Department of Acute Nursing Care, The University of Texas Health Science Center, San Antonio School of Nursing, 7703 Floyd Curl Drive, Mail Code 7975, San Antonio, TX 78229.

E-mail address: arevalol@uthscsa.edu

Perioperative Nursing Clinics 4 (2009) 287–296
doi:10.1016/j.cpen.2009.05.003 **periopnursing.theclinics.com**
1556-7931/09/$ – see front matter

Services in Health Care,[4] known as the CLAS Standards. These standards define cultural competence as follows:[4]

> *A set of congruent behaviors, attitudes, and policies that come together in a system, agency, or among professionals that enables effective work in cross-cultural situations. "Culture" refers to integrated patterns of human behavior that include the language, thoughts, communications, actions, customs, beliefs, values, and institutions of racial, ethnic, religious, or social groups. "Competence" implies having the capacity to function effectively as an individual and an organization within the context of the cultural beliefs, behaviors, and needs presented by consumers and their communities.*

Cultural competence can be defined as a long-term continuous process rather than an end product. It is "the ability to understand and constructively relate to the uniqueness of each [individual] in light of the diverse cultures that influence each person's perspective."[5] Central to the cultural competence process is the acknowledgment that there is value in it and that there must be continuous work toward culturally competent practices.[6]

FROM CULTURAL DESTRUCTIVES TO CULTURAL COMPETENCE

A commonly used and referenced model of the cultural competence process is the Cross model.[7,8] The model describes cultural competency as progress along a continuum that is based on the ability to respect and appreciate individual and cultural differences. Organizations and individuals can be at different stages of the continuum simultaneously. For instance, a researcher can be at the cultural precompetence stage in regard to recognizing racial, ethnic, and cultural differences but be at the cultural incapacity stage with reference to religious practices or sexual orientation. The model has six stages arranged in order of increasing competence: (1) cultural destructiveness, (2) cultural incapacity, (3) cultural blindness, (4) cultural precompetence, (5) cultural competence, and (6) cultural proficiency.

Cultural Destructiveness

Cultural destructiveness is the negative end of the continuum. In this stage cultural differences are viewed as a problem. Individuals believe that people should be more like the "mainstream" and assume that one culture is superior and should eradicate "lesser" cultures. The Tuskegee study is an example of this stage. This research was conducted on African American men to study the effects of syphilis when left untreated. The subjects were involved in this experiment without their knowledge or consent, currently accepted treatments were withheld, and participants were actively misled and given erroneous information.

Cultural Incapacity

Organizations and individuals in this stage lack cultural awareness and skills. Individuals may believe in the racial superiority of the dominant group and assume a paternalistic posture toward "lesser" groups. Research practices in this stage include maintaining stereotypes and the intentional and volitional exclusion of racial and ethnic minorities from research studies.

Cultural Blindness

In the middle of the continuum are individuals and organizations that believe that culture, race, or color make no difference. Individuals may see themselves as unbiased, but they do not perceive or benefit from the contributions and benefits of diverse populations. Scientists conducting research studies that include only white, middle class males may be in this stage. The exclusion of ethnic minorities at this stage is more an act of omission than an intentional exclusion. Not including women and racial minorities in clinical trials, for instance, has caused health care practitioners to prescribe drugs that may not have been tested on females or men of color.

Cultural Precompetence

Individuals in this stage recognize that there are cultural differences and begin to educate themselves and others about these differences; however, they may become complacent in their efforts. In this stage, organizations may attempt to address diversity issues by hiring a diverse staff and by offering cultural sensitivity training. Research at this stage is characterized by studies in which consents, recruiting materials, and instruments have been translated, and research team members speak the language spoken by the participants. Nevertheless, the study protocols may fail to accommodate cultural differences, or the data analysis does not include an examination of how the racial, ethnic, and cultural differences are related to the phenomenon under study.

Cultural Competence

Acceptance and respect of cultural differences characterizes this stage. Diversity is valued and cultural differences are accommodated. In addition, individuals accept the influence of their own culture in relation to other cultures. Research studies in this stage include ethnic and racial minorities, examine similarities between these groups, and explain whether differences between groups can be accounted for by biologic factors (eg, age, gender, and race) or sociocultural factors (eg, racism, poverty, immigration, cultural values). Research that is culturally competent aims at increasing the base of knowledge about a given aspect of a racial, ethnic, or minority group.

Cultural Proficiency

In this stage individuals and organizations move from accepting, appreciating, valuing, and accommodating cultural differences to an active stage in which others are educated about these differences. The knowledge gained from culturally competent research studies is integrated into a program of research that provides a wider theoretical and empiric knowledge base. This knowledge guides the design and implementation of programs and interventions aimed at improving the quality of life of culturally diverse groups.

THE BENEFIT OF CULTURALLY COMPETENT RESEARCH

Conducting culturally competent research studies generates knowledge that can lead to the transformation of beliefs, attitudes, and practices of those in charge of providing services to diverse communities. In no other area is this transformation more needed than in the delivery of health care services. The Institute of Medicine report *Unequal Treatment: Confronting Racial and Ethnic Disparities in Health Care*[3] states that racial and ethnic minorities tend to receive a lower quality of health care than nonminorities, even when access-related factors (eg, insurance and income) are taken into account. According to *Healthy People 2010*,[9] information available about the biologic and genetic characteristics of African Americans, Hispanics, American Indians, Alaska Natives, Asians, Native Hawaiians, and Pacific Islanders does not explain the health disparities experienced by these groups when compared with the white, non-Hispanic population in the United States. These disparities are thought to be the result of complex interactions among genetic variations, environmental factors, and specific health behaviors.[9]

The elimination of disparities in health care outcomes is a major challenge because the problem does not have a single cause. The barriers that separate individuals from quality health care include a lack of health information, comorbidities, attitudes about accessing health care, a shortage of health care providers, poverty, and cultural competency.[10] Although there is no unique manner to build cultural competency, conducting research that is culturally competent can generate the knowledge needed to address aspects of each of the barriers to quality care. Culturally competent research can help mitigate health disparities by generating the knowledge needed by providers to change their beliefs and practices to accommodate the unique needs of racial and ethnic minority populations.

WHAT DOES CULTURALLY COMPETENT RESEARCH LOOK LIKE?

Evaluating culturally competent research and scholarship can be facilitated by using eight criteria that guide the development of knowledge for culturally competent care and the determination of rigor and credibility in research with diverse, marginalized populations or populations in transitions.[11] These criteria, proposed by Meleis in 1996, are directed at all racial, ethnic, and cultural groups. In addition, the criteria focus on critical aspects of culture and interpersonal interactions across populations rather than on sections of the research process or report. The Meleis guidelines come close to "the dynamic, transactional, empowering process common to many definitions of cultural competence."[12] The eight criteria capture adequately the breadth of cultural competence in research. The criteria are contextuality, relevance, communication styles, awareness of identity and power differentials, disclosure, reciprocation, empowerment, and time.

Contextuality

Contextuality is the knowledge of research participants' lifestyles, situations, and the historical and sociopolitical conditions that affect them. The context is essential to develop the research questions and to understand the meaning of the results. Knowledge without a context can lead to stereotyping and marginalization of groups. Oakes and colleagues[13] provide an excellent example of contextuality in their description of the Hispanic population in the United States, the barriers that Hispanic Alzheimer's caregivers face, and the need to adapt previous existing programs for caregivers. The researchers in this study acknowledged early in the design that Hispanic caregiving might be different from that of any other group.

Reporting accurately the race, ethnicity, and nationality of research participants is also indicative of the researcher's effort to meet the criterion of contextuality. Although the definitions of ethnicity are as varied as the definitions of culture, the National Institutes of Health (NIH) recognize two ethnicities: (1) Hispanic or Latino and (2) non-Hispanic or Latino. A Hispanic individual can be of any race (white, black, Asian, native Hawaiian or other Pacific Islander, and American Indian or Alaskan native). Reporting the nationality (nativity) of the participants is also helpful given the different historical and sociopolitical conditions that affect different subgroups. For instance, Hispanics born in the United States may have different lifestyles and socioeconomic characteristics than Hispanics who have immigrated to the United States. Among the latter, immigrants from countries in South America may have different motives and forms of entry into the United States than Cubans.

In their study of differences in depression between Puerto Rican and non-Latina white mothers of adults with mental retardation, Magaña and colleagues[14] describe their research sample in a manner that is not misleading and denotes knowledge of subgroup differences:

> *The Puerto Rican sample consisted of 66 families who lived in Massachusetts. All the mothers were first-generation immigrants (95.5% were born in Puerto Rico), and all of the adults with mental retardation were of Puerto Rican descent. Two mothers were born in the Dominican Republic but lived in Puerto Rico for a period of time and had a spouse who was Puerto Rican. One mother was born in Colombia and had a spouse from Puerto Rico. On average, the mothers had lived in the United States for an average of 22.1 years at the time of the study.*

The researchers also included in the sample description the preferred language, recruitment methodology, and a contrast with the non-Latina sample of mothers.

Relevance

The criterion of relevance refers to whether the research questions serve a population's issues and interests in improving lives.[11] Evidence of establishing relevance in the research process can be obtained by reviewing the level of participation of the study population. For relevance, the research report must reflect how the formulation of questions, the interpretation of the data, and the dissemination of findings were informed and influenced by the community under study.

The discussion section on the significance of a research study for a population under study may show the weakness of meeting the criterion of relevance.[12] The significance may be clear to health care providers and scientists but not to members of the community. Stronger evidence is present when the population sees the topic of study as important in their lives, and when the significance of the study is explained to them using cultural knowledge.[12] The strongest evidence of relevance is present when the community requests or helps develop the research. Community-based participatory research (CBPR) studies are generally good examples of strong evidence of relevance. In this collaborative approach to scientific inquiry, researchers and community members are equal partners in the research process. CBPR starts with a research topic of interest to the community in a grass roots approach and aims at achieving social changes that improve the health care outcomes and quality of life of the community. In San Antonio, Texas, the program called "Familias en Acción" (Families in Action) is a 1.8 million dollar CBPR violence prevention NIH-funded study. Harlandale Independent School District (predominantly Hispanic) community members have made major decisions about the components of the study. In addition, about 20 trained community members collect the data. The principal investigators acknowledge that this approach makes sense because these community members know best what is happening in their neighborhoods.[15]

Communication Styles

Culturally competent research includes evidence of understanding the subtleties and variations in language and symbols.[11] The researcher must provide evidence of critical understanding of participants' preferred communication styles, language, and use and meaning of words. In addition, the researchers must provide evidence of knowledge and understanding of participants' familiarity with oral, written, and scaled responses.[12]

This criterion calls for much more than the translation of written materials or the use of bilingual interviewers. The researchers must convey in-depth understanding of language, meaning, and symbolisms that may hinder or enhance the research process. Appropriate translation and interpretation methodologies are crucial to show evidence of meeting the communication style criterion. Casually mentioning that the English version of an instrument was translated to the language preferred by the participants or that trained bilingual research team members collected data does not provide evidence of an in-depth understanding of language and meaning.

The most popular translation method is back-translation.[16,17] In this methodology, one person or a team translates the measures from the source language (most likely English) into the target language. Brislin[16,17] recommends extensive note taking during this process to identify terms that are difficult to translate or that require cultural rather than literal linguistic equivalence. Once this translation is finished, a different person or team translates the first version back to English. If there are discrepancies in the two versions, they are resolved through decentering. In this process, the researcher reads the back-translation to identify words that cannot be well translated and consults with a team of bilinguals (review committee) to revise the source language version. This process continues until there is evidence that cross-cultural equivalence has been obtained in regard to content, semantics, and conceptual equivalencies. Others have described the extensive process needed to assess the true psychometric estimates of any translated scale or instrument.[18] These processes go well beyond mere verbal translation and back-translation.

The dual-focus approach to translation[19] is derived from the distinction between emic (culture bound) and etic (universal) constructs. In constructing a translation, etic concepts are operationalized in each culture using emic concepts whose validity may be culture bound.[19] In this approach the following steps take place: (1) ethnic and nonethnic members of the research team define the problem for investigation, (2) the concepts to be studied are investigated from an etic and emic perspective, (3) specific items are created to measure these concepts, and (4) monolingual and bilingual focus groups are initiated to achieve the final translation of the measure. When the measure is finalized, its psychometric properties can be evaluated. With this methodology, English and the second language are both target languages, and the translators and members of the focus groups are major players in the study. This methodology is more time and labor intensive than back-translation.

As previously mentioned, casually mentioning in a research report that translators and interpreters were provided is not evidence of an in-depth knowledge of communication styles. The research reviewer and the participants must be able to clearly identify the level of knowledge of the research team members. Esposito[20] provides a description of a research team studying perimenopausal Hispanic women as follows:

> *The focus group team was made up of the principal investigator (PI), who is monolingual (English); one graduate research assistant (bilingual with English as a first language); the group facilitator (bilingual); and a professional translator. The college educated group facilitator was recruited from the community.*
>
> *Her command of local Spanish was obvious. Unfortunately, despite Spanish as her natal language, a bilingual upbringing, and use of Spanish in everyday life, she was educated in American schools, and her communication style did not reflect everyday language of those educated in a Spanish-speaking school system. This was revealed by some word confusion and slang that appeared in the transcripts.*
>
> *In contrast to the facilitator, who was a self-taught translator, the professional translator/interpreter completed postgraduate work in translation. She was credentialed by the United Nations and the US State Department to translate Spanish to English. In addition, she met the criteria for membership in the Translators and Interpreters Guild (1999), one of several professional organizations that provide standards for translation and interpretation.*

The above description provides reviewers with a clear picture of the language knowledge and skills of each of the research team members. Esposito[20] discusses issues of translation and interpretation and how they were handled to best ensure capturing the true meaning of the experience for the research participants.

Meaning

Central to the translation of scales and the collection and interpretation of data is the issue of meaning. Words in the language in which a scale is developed may not mean the same in another language. Culturally competent research reflects acknowledgment and exploration of these differences. The word "burden," for instance, has been translated to Spanish as the word "carga;" however, in the context of Hispanic/Latino family caregiving, the word carga is not appropriate.[21] Monolingual (Spanish) Hispanic/Latino caregivers of a relative with Alzheimer's disease, regardless of gender, relationship to the care receiver, number of years of caregiving, and perceived negative impact of caregiving, have been shown to deny experiencing carga or seeing their relative as a carga. For these Spanish-speaking caregivers, carga has various meanings including a heavy object, a weight, a sack, to be in charge of, paying attention to, something you carry or dispose of, a permanent bother, what is carried by trucks or animals, or something difficult and slaving.[21] Comparison of the perception of the experience of caregiving between monolingual and bilingual (English/Spanish) Latino/Hispanic caregivers of a relative with Alzheimer's disease[21] showed that cultural factors (values and beliefs) more than language alone determined the meaning and perception of the caregiving experience. Bilingual Latino/Hispanic caregivers also denied experiencing burden, seeing their duties as a burden, and thinking that their relative was a burden. Despite the existence of the word burden in their English vocabulary, the meaning of this word was equivalent to the descriptors used by the Spanish-speaking caregivers.

Awareness of Identity and Power Differential

A researcher and a participant can never possess equal power.[11] There is a distance created by knowledge, the purpose of the research encounter, identities, roles, and hierarchies. It is virtually impossible for the researcher and the participant to exercise the same degree of power. Evidence of the researcher's efforts to develop horizontal relationships rather than vertical differentiation satisfies this criterion. A common strategy in this direction is the use of community members to collect data.

Stronger evidence of an effort toward power equity is demonstrated in research studies in which the questions are generated by the community under study, and the data becomes the property of both the researcher and participants. At the University of Nebraska-Lincoln (UNL), the informed consent letters for Native American groups are allowed to have a more familiar symbol at the top of the letters. This symbol is approved by a local advisory board to represent the partnership between UNL and the tribes.[22] Native field researchers are trained in face-to-face sessions and not via the Internet. In addition, the UNL requests that the tribal council appoint an advisory board for the research project. UNL researchers restrict access to the data to project personnel, and the tribes are given the assurance that no one will merge tribal data with other data to make comparisons across racial groups, suggesting that certain problems may be more pervasive among American Indians. The tribes receive the summary of the research, and any research prepared for publication from a project is sent to the tribal advisory board before submission. If the board members raise any issues of cultural appropriateness of the research, UNL researchers review them and respond before submission for publication.[22]

Disclosure

To meet this criterion, researchers must demonstrate evidence of trust building.[11] Culturally competent research provides evidence of the strategies used to establish rapport and gain the trust of the participants. The job of the researcher is to uncover participants' experiences in a manner that is authentic to them and understandable to others.[11] The participants must be able to freely participate, respond, and disengage from the research process if they choose to do so. The privacy of the participants must be respected, and the research agenda, methods, and findings must be characterized by transparency. Secrecy has no place in culturally competent research.

Reciprocation

This criterion is achieved when the goals of the researcher and participants are identified and every attempt is made to ensure that these goals are met.[11] For some participants, the main goal may be to receive a financial incentive in exchange for participation. For other participants, the goal may be learning about their situation, answering questions, or improvement of their quality of life and that of their communities. The complete absence of reciprocation is illustrated by "helicopter research." This term refers to the old model of research in Indian country. In this type of study, researchers, often faculty from a university, would descend on the reservation to do research on Indians that might or might not address any needs of that community. Once data were collected, the researchers would fly away, never to be seen again.[23]

Empowerment

One of the tasks of the researcher is to construct credible descriptions of ways in which the research process has made or will make a contribution to the participants to increase control over their lives.[11] Participants in culturally competent research studies feel connected to the study and can exercise the freedom of making changes in their lives and in their communities.

Empowerment is especially important in research with marginalized populations. Through culturally competent research, marginalized cultural minorities can gain access to information and resources that enable them to learn skills, make choices, and become change agents. Empowerment must be at the core of research aimed at closing the gap in health care disparities.

Time

Culturally competent research is flexible in its approach to time.[11] This flexibility must be reflected in the time taken to gain the trust of the participants or the communities, to identify reciprocal goals, to plan actions, and to complete the research process. This criterion also calls for an understanding of how participants view time and for accommodations to address the participants' perspective of time.

Meeting this criterion presents a challenge. Although the researcher may strive for time flexibility in each step of the research process, organizational constraints and the guidelines of funding agencies may negatively impact the research timeline. Meleis[11] states that culturally competent research is not constrained by time or by an exact number of research-participant encounters. Furthermore, the consistency of time between participants and interviewers and consistency in the number of interviews may be sacrificed for reciprocity, empowerment, and disclosure.[11]

SUMMARY

This article has provided an overview of the stages in the Cross[7,8] continuum of cultural competency and has described Meleis'[11] eight cultural competence guidelines for research. Culturally competent research presents several challenges. In fact, it may be unrealistic to expect any single researcher to become an expert in working with cultural, racial, ethnic, and minority populations. Team and collaborative research efforts might make meeting the goal of cultural competence more realistic. It is also unrealistic to expect that every study conducted with culturally diverse populations will meet prospectively or retrospectively all of the criteria formulated by Meleis.[11] Conducting research that is culturally competent contributes to our progress as a society toward a stage of cultural proficiency. Researchers striving to conduct studies that meet Meleis'[11] criteria for cultural competence contribute to the generation of the knowledge needed to close the gap in health disparities.

ACKNOWLEDGMENTS

The author wishes to thank The John A. Hartford Foundation Building Academic Geriatric Nursing Capacity Program for its support during the preparation of this article. Special thanks to Michael Sierra-Arévalo for his thoughtful comments.

REFERENCES

1. US Census Bureau. An older and more diverse nation by midcentury. Available at: http://www.census.gov/Press-Release/www/releases/archives/population/012496.html. Accessed March 10, 2009.
2. US Department of Health and Human Services. Health disparities–closing the gap fact sheet. Available at: http://ncmhd.nih.gov/hdFactSheet_gap.asp. National Center on Minority Health and Health Disparities. Accessed March 10, 2009.
3. Smedley BD, Stith AY, Nelson AR, editors. Unequal treatment: confronting racial and ethnic disparities in health care. Institute of Medicine. Washington, DC: National Academies Press; 2003.
4. US Department of Health and Human Services. National standards for cultural and linguistically appropriate services in health care: final report. US Department of Health and Human Services Office of Minority Health. Available at: http://www.omhrc.gov/assets/pdf/checked/finalreport.pdf. Accessed February 20, 2009.
5. Stuart R. Twelve practical suggestions for achieving multicultural competence. Prof Psychol Res Pr 2004;35:3–9.
6. Reich SM, Reich JA. Cultural competence in interdisciplinary collaborations: a method for respecting diversity in research partnerships. Am J Community Psychol 2006;38:51–62.
7. Cross T. Services to minority populations: cultural competence continuum. Focal Point 1988;3(1):1–4.
8. Cross T, Bazron B, Dennis K, et al. Towards a culturally competent system of care vol. 1. Washington, DC: Georgetown University Child Development Center, CASSP Technical Assistance Center; 1989.
9. US Department of Health and Human Services. Healthy people 2010. 2nd edition. Washington (DC): US Government Printing Office; 2000.
10. US Department of Health and Human Services. HRSA care action. Providing HIV/AIDS care in a changing environment. Mitigating health disparities through

cultural competence. HRSA Care Action August 2002. Available at: http://hab.hrsa.gov.
11. Meleis AI. Culturally competent scholarship: substance and rigor. Adv Nurs Sci 1996;19:1–16.
12. Jacobson SF, Chu NL, Pascucci MA, et al. Culturally competent scholarship in nursing research. J Transcult Nurs 2005;16:202–9.
13. Oakes SL, Hepburn K, Silva Ross J, et al. Reaching the heart of the caregiver. Clin Gerontol 2006;30:37–49.
14. Magaña S, Seltzer M, Wyngaarden KM. Cultural context of caregiving: differences in depression between Puerto Rican and non-Latina white mothers of adults with mental retardation. Ment Retard 2004;42:1–11.
15. Martinez MM. Harlandale residents to research violence. My SAnews. Available at: http://www.mysanantonio.com/news/MYSA050906_3B_violenceprevention_120cc176_html9049.html. Accessed March 10, 2009.
16. Brislin RW. Back-translation for cross-cultural research. J Cross Cult Psychol 1970;1:185–216.
17. Brisling RW. The wording and translation of research instruments. In: Lonner WJ, Brislin RW, editors. Cross-cultural research methods. New York: Wiley; 1973. p. 137–65.
18. Froman RD, Owen SV. Instrumentation concerns for multicultural research. In: The nursing profession: tomorrow and beyond. Thousand Oaks (CA): Sage; 2001. p. 397–405.
19. Erkut S, Alarcón O, García Coll C, et al. The dual-focus approach to creating bilingual measures. J Cross Cult Psychol 1999;30:206–18.
20. Esposito N. From meaning to meaning: the influence of translation techniques of non-English focus group research. Qual Health Res 2001;11:568–79.
21. L.C. Arévalo-Flechas. Factors influencing Latino/Hispanic caregivers' perception of the experience of caring for a relative with Alzheimers disease. Available at: http://proquest.umi.com/pqdweb?did=1564020851&sid=1&Fmt=6&clientId=70986&RQT=309&VName=PQD.
22. Vasgird D. Making research trustworthy for Native Americans. Empir Res Hum Res Ethics 2007;2:84–5.
23. Grim CW. Indian health service research program, policy, and priorities. Indian Health Service. Available at: http://www.ihs.gov/publicinfo/publicaffairs/director/2006_statements/ihs_research_conference-april_24-word-version-web.pdf. Accessed March 9, 2009.

Dissemination of Findings: The Final Step of Investigation

Nancy Girard, PhD, RN, FAAN

KEYWORDS

- Quality improvement • Research • Publication
- Writing • Publication

The final step in any investigative process is the dissemination of the information and knowledge gained from the findings. This reporting is essential for the growth of individuals, the care for the patient, and the forward movement of the nursing profession. Although the final outcome of the research process more often incorporates publication than does the Quality Improvement (QI) process, it is vital that results and findings from every area be considered by practitioners to gather the best evidence for practice.

This article discusses the importance of publication; explores the differences between the manuscripts for research and QI, and characteristics of both; and provides writing tips related to preparing a manuscript for publication.

IMPORTANCE OF PUBLISHING FINDINGS

Why publish research or QI work? The answer is that information, to be useful, must be available to all potential users. Only when there is close scrutiny by others of the problem presented, methods used in investigation, data collection, analysis and interpretation, can the information be determined to be useful. When there are questions, equivocation, or controversy involving the outcomes, dialog is vital to develop useable knowledge. Indeed, the old saying, "the study isn't done until it is published" is true. Knowledge must be shared. How many clinicians have spent considerable time, even years, on solving a problem in our institution, then have found out others had the same problem and had solved it? The nursing profession cannot continue to grow without concepts being tested, theories being questioned, and practice being improved.

The publication of outcomes from QI or research projects benefits patients. The benefits of a QI study can result in immediate safety improvement in patient care.

Department of Acute Nursing Care, University of Texas Health Science Center School of Nursing, 7703 Floyd Curl Drive, San Antonio, TX 78229, USA
E-mail address: ngirard2@satx.rr.com

Perioperative Nursing Clinics 4 (2009) 297–306
doi:10.1016/j.cpen.2009.05.009 **periopnursing.theclinics.com**

Research findings can also affect patient care, benefiting them directly or indirectly as the translation to practice continues to improve.

Publication also benefits the author and his or her organization. If the organization is a hospital going for "magnet status", publication of QI projects demonstrates that the activity and quality of the nurses and the emphasis on continuing improvement of the organization. It also helps nurses directly when they are going for promotion on a clinical ladder and helps them with eligibility for certification. If one is associated with an educational institution, he or she must publish to show academic activity and to be promoted. Some universities require publication by full-time faculty and include this in the decision to offer tenure or post-tenure appointment.

Whether research or QI, there are many ways that knowledge can be shared. Presentations, poster sessions, written reports, and publication of manuscripts are the most common ways. Most agree that the hardest part is the writing of the study. If an oral podium presentation or poster has been completed and the information shared, then that study can still be submitted for publication. If the poster has been published in a conference handout, then that information can, and should, be referenced in a formal manuscript when submitting to a journal.

DIFFERENCES BETWEEN QUALITY IMPROVEMENT AND RESEARCH

The differences between research and QI projects are often unclear to those not closely involved with either type of study. Three main differences exist: the projects' intent and purposes differ; they differ in generalizability; and they often show different associated risks to subjects.[1]

The intent and purpose of research is to generate new knowledge or test theories; QI examines an internal process of a specific institution to improve practice (**Table 1**). Both use the scientific method, involving generating a question or identifying a problem, planning methods of investigation, collecting data, analyzing data and interpreting results. The same or similar approach is used in both with a difference in emphasis on control. QI projects often take place in a single institution, while empiric research can be done in multiple clinical sites. In the single site application of QI, there is often more control. When multiple sites are used, it is very difficult to control all the variables and rule out any extraneous influence because site-specific factors may affect findings. To address this concern, there is specific emphasis in research to control as many variables as possible to make results more interpretable. Unlike

Table 1
Comparison of research and quality improvement

Research	Quality Improvement
1. Generates new knowledge or tests theories	1. Examines an process internal to an organization to improve care
2. Results potentially generalizable to other settings and individuals	2. Results usually primarily valid in study institution
3. Emphasis on control of variables	3. Emphasis on delivery of care processes rather than control
4. Participants are representative of the population of interest	4. Participants are in institution (employees or patients) invited to participate
5. May pose risks to participants; requires approval from review board or ethics committee with consent to participate	5. Low, if any, risk to participants; may or may not have to get ethics committee approval

research applications, QI does not usually attempt such strict control of variables in a project, but instead it emphasizes ways to improve the delivery of care.

The difference in number of sites used, or population addressed, is the source of the second distinction between research and QI. With research, results are more likely to be generalizable to other settings; in contrast, QI findings may be specific to the one setting where a project was implemented and findings are pertinent only to that setting. In QI projects, personnel in the setting are included or invited to be part of the investigation. QI projects are often implemented by nurses who have identified a problem with patient care within a hospital or unit. Depending on the type of QI project, approval may be required from a hospital committee, ethics committee, or oversight group.[2] With research, the sample of participants is from a population of interest that is not necessarily tied to any one institution and is defined with very clear and specific criteria for inclusion and exclusion. For example, a research study of thermal regulation of postoperative patients might be conducted in any institution, but the research would need to identify age, surgical type, comorbid conditions, and other criteria that might need to be met for inclusion as a participant.

Research must be approved by an institutional review board (IRB) and requires written consent of the subjects to participate. The IRB assesses the potential risk and commensurate benefit to patients as participants, safe-guarding their rights. QI might not have to meet those requirements for IRB approval and consent because QI does not generally pose risks to patient participants.

CHARACTERISTICS OF A RESEARCH STUDY

Research studies pose specific questions for inquiry or hypotheses to be tested to advance science and general knowledge. There are various types of research, including both qualitative and quantitative approaches, which show differing characteristics and approaches. The articles in this volume by Beck (qualitative) and by Holtzclaw (quantitative) provide extensive descriptions of the two types of research approaches. The interested reader is directed to those articles for descriptions of the characteristics of those studies.

CHARACTERISTICS OF A QI STUDY

A QI project is designed to improve delivery, efficiency, or outcome of patient care or service provided. The findings contribute to the evidence used in developing best clinical practices. The methodical process of investigation is usually used in the identification of quality indicators and measures used.[3]

Although there are various methods used in QI, one of the most common methods is a process that plans, collects data, analyzes the findings, evaluates the outcomes and acts to implement a revised or new tool or procedure. With planning, the problem is identified, the people or process involved solicited, and a data collection protocol is developed. The process decided upon is then implemented for a specific length of time and the data collected and analyzed. Action is then taken if results indicate a method for improvement, the action is evaluated, and a revised or new process is implemented.

WRITING AND PUBLICATION TIPS

Choosing the Correct Journal

It helps publication efforts if the author chooses the correct journal for submission of a manuscript (electronic or hard copy). There is a wide selection of journals available today for authors. Indeed, a search online for nursing journals shows close to 300 electronic and traditional format journals worldwide, all of which are interested in receiving manuscripts. The choice of a journal in which to publish one's study depends upon the content of the manuscript, the type of study, the focus of the journal, and the need of the author(s) to publish in a certain journal. Electronic publications have a very quick turn-around and manuscripts have the potential to be published within weeks of being submitted. Manuscripts submitted to traditional print journals, depending on the popularity and competitive nature of the journal, can take 6 months to 2 years to be seen in print. Most journals will require written statements of conflict of interest, association with business or industry, and copyright when manuscripts are received. Recently, some journal editors began requiring forms declaring authorship contribution and other forms that would protect the journal against articles containing deliberately wrong analysis and data from research. These procedures are being introduced because the editors of some prestigious medical journal have been fired because of publication of research containing fictitious or wrong data and interpretation.

Publication in research journals is an expectation for nurses in academia. There are many excellent journals that focus on research, such as *Western Journal of Nursing Research* or *Research in Nursing & Health*. These journals are very prestigious for academicians who seek to publish in journals that are highly regarded as competitive and that carry a high impact factor These journals prefer well-controlled, well-executed, qualitative and quantitative research and they are very prescriptive in criteria for acceptance. They typically have submitted manuscripts reviewed by a number of experts to assess quality and potential to contribute to theory or practice. These journals frequently request revisions, clarifications, or additions to submitted manuscripts during the review process. It is not unknown to receive two or more pages describing questions, edits, points needing clarification, or changes before acceptance of a manuscript for publication. Research, to be useful to practitioners and the nursing profession, must be good science.

Clinical journals also publish research of interest to their readers, and the editors look for well-done QI project reports. Recently, the focus of clinical journals began to more heavily emphasize articles that support evidence for practice and patient safety, reflecting the prevailing evidence-based practice Zeitgeist. Specialty organizations that produce their own journal, such as perioperative nursing (AORN Journal), critical care, orthopedic nursing, are excellent journals and they are always looking for manuscripts. Articles reflecting the specialty are especially welcome, as are articles about topics that can be associated with any care, such as geriatric patients, communication needs, and leadership.

Some journals reflect nursing in general, such as the American Journal of Nursing. They accept manuscripts that contain information on a variety of topics, including theory, research, QI, clinical, leadership and educational practices. All the above journals solicit manuscripts and accept unsolicited manuscripts for review as well.

Other journals, such as Perioperative Nursing Clinics, are topic or planned journal issues, such as this one, and selectively appoint authors to write on a topic already specified. Unsolicited manuscripts usually are not accepted unless the manuscript is specifically on the topic designated for a planned volume. It is best to look at upcoming issue plans to see the monthly topics, and then contact the editor to see if a manuscript is needed. An email or letter to the editor before submitting the manuscript will save time and energy if the journal does not want or need an article such as the one proposed.

Authors in nursing should consider general layman publications because the dissemination on knowledge should include those people whom nurses are always trying to teach, inform and protect. This area is very much ignored today. Physicians do a much better job of educating the public than do nurses, who tend to share knowledge with only their own.

Choosing the correct journal in advance will help target an audience and determine the format, writing style and emphasis for a manuscript, and should be done in advance of constructing the manuscript. Selecting the appropriate journal will ensure the best chance of acceptance of an article. No matter which journal is targeted, requests for changes are not equivalent to a rejection of the manuscript. If rejected, the author will immediately get a letter saying so. If the manuscript is deemed salvageable, then a revision letter is sent. The majority of articles are not accepted without some revision; most are accepted following accurate and clear changes.

Deciding Credit of Authors

It is important to decide on authorship if there will be more than one, before beginning writing. If there are to be two or more authors, the ranking of names should also be decided, that is, who will be first and second author. The work of writing should also be determined at this time. It is helpful to have explicit deadlines for when written components of the manuscript should be ready and shared with the authoring team so that delays in progress do not occur.

All persons listed as authors must take responsibility for understanding the components of the full article and the contents therein. This requirement is common for both journals and professional organizations like AORN and the American Psychological Association. The *International Committee of Medical Journal Editors* specifically recommends that:[4]

> *"Each author make direct and substantial contributions in the conception and design of the study or project or data analysis and interpretation, AND in the drafting the article or revising it critically for important intellectual content, AND be able and willing to give final approval of the version to be published and to take public responsibility for the entire work."*

Most editors are using these or similar guidelines. No one should be listed as an author unless active and full participation has been contributed. For example, a person who has been consulted about content yet has not been active in the writing should be recognized in at the beginning or end or the article but not listed as an author. A faculty instructor overseeing a QI project for a course is performing his or her teaching duties and can also be given credit and recognition in an acknowledgment, but such as person should not be listed as an author. General recommendations are that no more than five authors should be listed on an article. This varies from journal to journal, and is generally clarified in the journal's author guidelines.

What to Include in Article

Most journals have a page limit for manuscripts. They will not accept a submission that is 50 plus pages long. Check journal guidelines for both length and style requirements. After being given length restrictions, the first thing that must be accomplished is shortening the paper to a limit imposed by the journal. Regardless of which journal a manuscript is submitted to, dissertations or theses must be changed from a formal school paper into a readable manuscript following journal specifications. The body of the paper must condense information and focus on the problem to be solved or question to be answered, the findings, the Implications for practice, education, and future research. Often, translating theses and dissertations into publishable manuscripts

Box 1
Checklist for submitting a research paper for publication

Always refer first to the journal's guidelines for authors and follow directions exactly

Title page

- ☐ The title includes the most important key word(s)
- ☐ Names of all authors with all full names and highest degrees (can add other credentials, depending on journal)
- ☐ Contact author's complete information
- ☐ State any grant support or business association
- ☐ Running head on all pages (2–5 words)

Abstract

- ☐ On its own page
- ☐ 150–350 words
- ☐ First sentence on what the article covers
- ☐ State the principal aims, instruments, and scope of paper or investigation
- ☐ Summarize the results or points

Introduction: new page to start body of the paper

- ☐ What the paper is about; problem or paper focus.
- ☐ Short, pertinent literature review
- ☐ Theory or concepts used and how this study will expand or build on present knowledge
- ☐ State the type of study, aims/research questions or hypotheses
- ☐ Identify outcomes or endpoints.
- ☐ Numbers on every page (eg, 1 of 1)

Body/methodology section

- ☐ Description of exact details, sources, methods or preparation
- ☐ Detailed description of interventions or treatment if used
- ☐ Identify populations, protection of subjects, criteria for inclusion and exclusion, and how number was determined
- ☐ Specification and definition for each variable
- ☐ Types of instruments used and validation/reliability information for each.
- ☐ Identify type of data analysis
- ☐ Clear and logical flow between ideas, paragraphs, sections
- ☐ Subheadings for new sections

Results/conclusion section

- ☐ Avoid jargon
- ☐ Speak to every aim/question/purpose identified in the introduction and findings for each
- ☐ Include all pertinent data. (If data is given in tables, don't repeat in words)
- ☐ Use only meaningful tables, graphs and statistics
- ☐ Avoid unnecessary repetition of information in both text and graphs
- ☐ Prepare all illustrations, tables, and graphs exactly as stated in editorial guidelines.

Discussion Section

- ☐ Interpret findings for readers. Were aims met? Research questions answered?
- ☐ Point out exceptions; define unsettled points; identify discrepancies and limitations
- ☐ Identify how experience/project/study agrees or disagrees with past findings/experience
- ☐ State conclusions clearly; do not overinterpret if findings not there
- ☐ Identify implications for practice
- ☐ Point out areas for further practice/study/research

Acknowledgments and references

- ☐ Recognize grant support
- ☐ Acknowledge persons contributing to paper who are not authors
- ☐ Check references for accuracy and conforming to journal format
- ☐ Check that Web references are still available and correct

Illustrations, graphs, tables, and figures

- ☐ List on separate page
- ☐ Give number, legend for each
- ☐ Be sure that each is referenced in the textual narrative.

means there should be less content on the conceptual framework and background, and a streamlined literature review.

If the article is a research article, a brief description of the theoretical or conceptual framework will often suffice. There also must be evidence of protection of subjects (IRB approval), methods, instruments, sampling, results, and discussion. References for a journal article can also be condensed by shortening the background and literature review. Data should be included that explain the whole study and the findings.[5]

A checklist for suggestions in what to include is a research article can be seen in **Box 1**.

If it is impossible to shorten the manuscript because of the topic of the study, check with the editor in advance of complete preparation. It may be possible to write the manuscript in part I and part II sections. Different components of a research study can be presented however, such as a separate paper of methodology and one on the study findings. Finally, authors should be aware that most journals do not publish pilot studies, so the manuscript could be revised to read as literature review, problem identification or some other presentation other than as a pilot study. Most editors will request authors wait until the complete study is accomplished rather than publishing a pilot.

For QI projects, similar comments can be applied when writing up the study. A checklist for QI papers can be seen in **Box 2**.

Using Figures and Tables

Use of tables, figures and illustrations should be included in articles, and clear, descriptive legends must accompany them. Nothing is more confusing than to see a table with a large amount of data that are not identified and that are therefore uninterpretable. Some data can be eliminated from tables if the narrative contains the information. For example, if the paper discusses the subject demographics, it is

Box 2
Checklist for submitting a quality improvement article for publication

Always refer first to the journal's guidelines for authors and follow directions exactly

Title

- ☐ State main word/idea in title

Introduction

- ☐ Identified problem in study institution and why QI undertaken
- ☐ State study question and how it was investigated
- ☐ Overview evidence presently existing for best care
- ☐ Present what was to be achieved

Methods

- ☐ Setting
- ☐ Who participated and how
- ☐ How did planning progress and what was length of time of project
- ☐ What exactly was studied and how was study conducted (Can someone else do this QI project?)
- ☐ If pertinent, show how privacy concerns, HIPPA and other concerns were addressed
- ☐ What tests, instruments, measurements or counts were used
- ☐ How data were collected and analyzed

Outcomes

- ☐ Was care improved or problem minimized?
- ☐ What were the costs/benefits of change?
- ☐ What was learned and what would be done differently in future
- ☐ Barriers, boundaries and facilitators identified
- ☐ How do findings add to evidence for practice?

Summary

- ☐ What was done, why and usefulness of study
- ☐ Implications for nursing/patient care

References/resources

- ☐ Recognize grant or industry support
- ☐ Acknowledge persons contributing to paper who are not authors
- ☐ Check references for accuracy and conforming to journal format
- ☐ Check that Web references still available and correct.

unnecessary to also include that information in a table. In most cases of data, however, tables offer the most efficient means of presentation. If data are tabulated, then repetition of the same data in the narrative is unnecessary. All tables, graphs, and figures that are included in a manuscript should be referred to someplace in the narrative text so that readers know when best to consult those presentations. If possible, it is more pleasing to see a variety of tables. Bar or pie graphs should be included along with the usual tables because they provide more reader interest and can be used to focus the eye on parts of the study that might otherwise be just be ignored. This is especially useful in QI projects, which may not have as much formal, interval data.

Manuscript Problems

It should not have to be mentioned to a professional author, but every paper must have a beginning, middle and an end. Unfortunately, editors receive poorly written papers much too frequently. If the paper is too confusing, it will simply be rejected. With a multitude of papers coming in to the journal offices, editors do not have the time or patience to read a defectively written article.

Authors must be aware of the flow of information, grammar, sentence, and paragraph construction, and avoid the overuse of jargon. Nurses have been educated since day one to speak "nursesse." Jargon can be specific to the specialty practice area, and it can baffle a reader. Some words are totally overused today, or selected to be pseudo-sophisticated. One such pseudo-sophisticated word is "utilize" when the simple "use" will suffice. Jargon and excessive words should be kept to a minimum in writing.

Although computers are wonderfully helpful writing assistants, they can only do so much to help. If a word is misspelled, the computer can automatically correct it, but it might not be the word intended by the author. Therefore, close scrutiny to every word in the manuscript should occur before submission.

Do a final check of references. References used should be valid and up to date. Often a study takes a considerable amount of time and the references may not be available on the Web any longer. It will delay publication if these need to be updated. With the change of century, it is easy for a reviewer or editor to scan a reference list and see if the majority are studies published before 2000 and thus, now, at least a decade old and potentially out-of-date. Many journals require that references be 5 years or less old. Check with author guidelines for specific information on references. References older than 5–8 years may be accepted if they are classic articles, or the only ones existing. Be sure that references are primary references and not second- or third-hand reports. Textbooks should never be used as reference as they are all second-hand and probably over 5 years old by the time the book comes to publication.

Required Permits for Publication

Each journal will have required forms for publication submission. With electronic submissions, many forms are built into the process and may not be a separate form. An example of electronic information for potential authors can be seen on the Elsevier Web site at http://www.elsevier.com/wps/find/authorshome.authors. Author directions, submission directions and many other helpful details are found there. Other publishers have similar electronic submission sites, which can be determined by the journal for which one wants to write. With hard copy journals, author information is included in every issue, with detailed directions on how and what to submit.

As previously discussed, forms can be: copyright forms, as well as payment, conflict of interest, author determination, research verification, and permission to copy other works. All forms must be completed and in the hands of the publisher before an article goes to print.

SUMMARY

In conclusion, it is vital that both research and QI projects be shared through writing and publication. A work is not done until it is shared with others. There are differences in requirements for publication of each type of project, but both research and QI are worthy and vital in identifying and finding evidence for best practices. Indeed, both are needed to determine the best nursing care practices for today.

Reports of both research and QI should identify the next step or stage in growth, such as future research needed as identified in the study, or how the QI project identified research needed to find further answers in patient care. This discussion by authors often engages the reader in similar or subsequent research and QI efforts.

Finally, if nurses have taken the considerable time and effort to do either research or QI, their efforts must be recognized by peers and others, and this recognition can only be done through publication of those efforts.

REFERENCES

1. Cosco Theodore D, Alana Knopp BA, Milke Doris L. Investigative first steps: appropriate identification and ethical review of research and quality improvement. Available at: http://ojni.org/11_3/cosco.htm. Accessed April 1, 2009.
2. Morris Peter E, Dracup Kathleen. Quality improvement or research? The ethics of hospital project oversight (editorial). Am J Crit Care 2007;16:424–6. Available at: http://ajcc.aacnjournals.org/cgi/content/full/16/5/424. Accessed April 1, 2009.
3. The SQUIRE (Standards for Quality Improvement Reporting Excellence) guidelines for quality improvement reporting: explanation and elaboration. Qual Saf Health Care 2008;17(Suppl 1):i13–32. doi:10.1136/qshc.2008.029058. Published online 2008 September 26. Available at: http://www.pubmedcentral.nih.gov/articlerender.fcgi?artid=2602740. Accessed April 1, 2009.
4. International Committee of Medical Journal Editors. Uniform requirements for manuscripts submitted to biomedical journals: writing and editing for biomedical publication. Updated October 2008. Available at: http://www.icmje.org/. Accessed April 1, 2009.
5. Guidelines for Writing Scientific Papers. Available at: http://www.bms.bc.ca/library/Guidelines%20for%20writing%20Scientific%20papers.pdf. Accessed April 1, 2009.

Index

Note: Page numbers of article titles are in **boldface** type.

Perioperative Nursing Clinics 4 (2009) 307–315
doi:10.1016/S1556-7931(09)00059-X

R

S

V

W

Printed and bound by CPI Group (UK) Ltd, Croydon, CR0 4YY
03/10/2024
01040465-0011